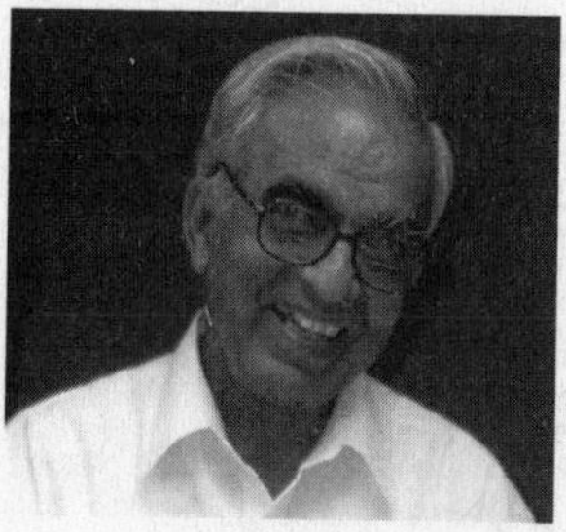

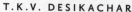

T.K.V. DESIKACHAR

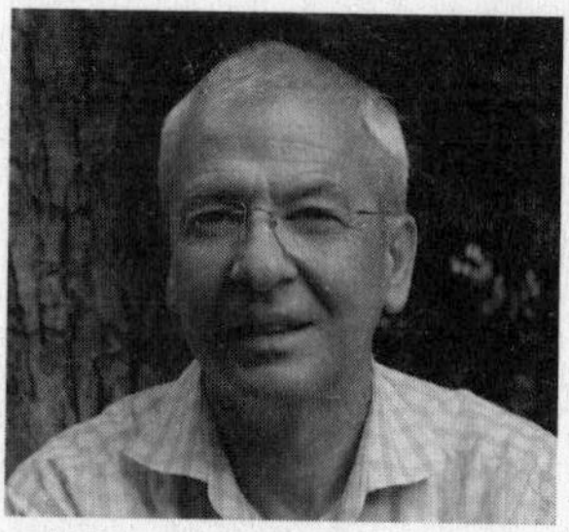

HELLFRIED KRUSCHE

FREUD AND YOGA

Translated by Anne-Marie Hodges

T.K.V. DESIKACHAR, son and longtime student of T. Krishnamacharya, is one of the world's foremost teachers of yoga. Born in Mysore in 1938, Desikachar became a renowned authority on the therapeutic uses of yoga and, in 1976, founded the Krishnamacharya Yoga Mandiram in Chennai, India. Desikachar withdrew from active teaching in 2013.

HELLFRIED KRUSCHE is a psychotherapist and psychoanalyst. He is a training analyst and supervisor for the International Psychoanalytical Association in Germany and lectures widely in Europe and Great Britain on yoga and psychoanalysis. Born in Aachen in 1951, he lives in Cologne, where he has a private practice.

ALSO BY T.K.V. DESIKACHAR

Health, Healing, and Beyond

The Heart of Yoga

The Viniyoga of Yoga

What We Are Seeking (with Martyn Neal)

Yoga Makaranda (with T. Krishnamacharya)

FREUD
and
YOGA

FREUD and YOGA

TWO PHILOSOPHIES OF MIND COMPARED

T.K.V. DESIKACHAR
AND HELLFRIED KRUSCHE

TRANSLATED FROM THE GERMAN BY
ANNE-MARIE HODGES

NORTH POINT PRESS
A division of Farrar, Straus and Giroux New York

North Point Press
A division of Farrar, Straus and Giroux
18 West 18th Street, New York 10011

Printed in the United States of America
Originally published in German, in slightly different form,
in 2007 by Theseus-Verlag, Germany,
as *Das verborgene Wissen bei Freud und Patañjali*
English translation published in the United States by North Point Press
First American edition, 2014

Library of Congress Cataloging-in-Publication Data
Desikachar, T.K.V., author.
[Verborgene Wissen bei Freud und Patañjali. English]
Freud and yoga : two philosophies of mind compared / T.K.V. Desikachar and Hellfried Krusche ; translated from the German by Anne-Marie Hodges. — First American edition.
pages cm
ISBN 978-0-86547-759-9 (paperback) — ISBN 978-0-86547-760-5 (ebook)
1. Mind and body. 2. Yoga. 3. Psychology. 4. Freud, Sigmund, 1856–1939. 5. Patañjali. I. Krusche, Hellfried. II. Title.

BF161 .D45513 2014
150.19'52—dc23

2014016951

Designed by Abby Kagan

www.fsgbooks.com
www.twitter.com/fsgbooks • www.facebook.com/fsgbooks

1 3 5 7 9 10 8 6 4 2

CONTENTS

PREFACE:
ON THE ORIGINS OF THIS BOOK

BY HELLFRIED KRUSCHE

This book is the result of a series of discussions with the yoga master T.K.V. Desikachar, son and student of the famous T. Krishnamacharya, one of the forefathers of yoga in the modern world.

After spending a seven-year period of intense training with his teacher in the Himalayas, Krishnamacharya lived for more than sixty years in southern India. His life's work led to the rediscovery of yoga and its many modern applications in the world today. Krishnamacharya's students, such as Pattabhi Jois, B.K.S. Iyengar, and above all his son, T.K.V. Desikachar, brought his authentic and yet individually adaptive form of yoga to the Western world and established it as an integral part of Western cultural life today.

Krishnamacharya was not only a yogi and a yoga teacher, he was also a poet, a singer, and an accomplished writer. He composed poems, sang Vedic hymns, and interpreted and commented on the Yogasūtra. Even less well known is that he was also a healer with in-depth knowledge of Ayurvedic medicine. An essential element of his wisdom was this unique combination of yoga and the traditional Vedic healing arts. For more than thirty years he imparted this knowledge and experience to his son and student, T.K.V. Desikachar.

In my conversations with T.K.V. Desikachar, we focused on those factors that play an active role in treatment and healing according to the perspective of traditional yoga. While doing this, we compared treatment models from classical psychoanalysis in dealing with psychological problems in a Western cultural context. We thus discussed differences between Eastern and Western approaches when dealing with illness and healing.

During one of our discussions, T.K.V. Desikachar expressed his wish that this dialogue be made available to a wider audience. It then also became clear that we would need to establish a basis to familiarize readers with essential terms and ideas from both yoga and psychoanalysis so that they could follow these discussions. We soon discovered surprising similarities in both approaches concerning the development and change of the psyche, which led in turn to this book.

In this context, T.K.V. Desikachar presents yoga according to the traditional teachings of Patañjali's Yogasūtra. This sutra text, approximately two thousand years old, with its numerous interpretations represents the philosophical foundation of yoga.

The English versions of the sutras in this text are based on T.K.V. Desikachar's translations as published in *The Heart of Yoga*. Based on my understanding as a psychotherapist trained in classical Freudian psychoanalysis, I conducted a dialogue with T.K.V. Desikachar on each sutra to understand his interpretation within the perspective of psychoanalysis.

These discussions took place over the course of a number of visits to Chennai, India, between 2000 and 2005. During this time, we were able to engage in a dialogue between two very different cultures about the methods employed by each culture to develop and change human experience and behavior. The result was a fascinating exchange on at times similar, at times different, approaches to health, development, consciousness, and freedom.

Yoga and psychoanalysis are proven techniques that can help people to develop. Both disciplines arose in separate cultures without influencing each other. Nonetheless, there are surprising similarities in certain areas and assumptions regarding basic psychological processes.

Yoga and psychoanalysis come to life through dialogue. In yoga, this is the dialogue between teacher and student; in psychoanalysis, it is the dialogue between psychoanalyst and patient. Following these traditions, we have kept this book in the form of a dialogue.

Dear reader, I hope that when reading this book you can enter into this living dialogue and that it transmits a helpful, practical notion of both yoga and psychoanalysis.

FREUD
and
YOGA

Introduction

BY HELLFRIED KRUSCHE

HEALING AND DEVELOPMENT

Across all cultures, people have always tried to enhance their psychological development with the help of spiritual and physical exercises and rituals. The search for ways to support spiritual transformation is ancient. Those vested with the secrets of such development and transformation were usually priests. They managed this sacred knowledge, which they felt came directly from a divine source, and therefore controlled secret information that also enabled health and healing. Philosophy and medicine were thus connected by their common divine and cultic origins.

In the Western world, we see an example of this in ancient Greece in Epidaurus, where the demigod Asclepius, son of Apollo, was said to have treated and healed as a doctor within a religious, cultic setting in the fifth century B.C.E. Methods attributed to him involved ritual cleansing, baths, healing sleep, and dream analysis. Dreams were thought to have been messages from the gods and were thus treated seriously and interpreted in dialogue with the priest/doctor. Participation in cultural events, especially theater productions, was felt to help free blocked emotions, and the resulting feelings and identification were thought to enable new insights. Releasing emotions helped to heal the soul through the process of catharsis.

Thus, treatments of this sort were initially holistic. They dealt with both physical and emotional aspects of well-being. An important foundation for practicing this kind of healing was the correct interpretation of secret messages from the gods, which were revealed to people in their dreams. The understanding of these messages was derived through the discussions people had with their doctors, who were also priests of the demigod Asclepius.

PSYCHOANALYSIS

In the modern world, philosophy, the natural sciences, and theology have all become separate disciplines. Medicine became one of the natural sciences and later came to include psychoanalysis as a means of treating mental disorders. Psychoanalysis is considered the foundation for most forms of psychotherapy. Sigmund Freud, a doctor of medicine and a neurologist, had also been educated in philosophy. He recognized neuroses as a developmental dysfunction in the human psyche. By devising a way to help patients represent their inner world in language and then again use words to solve their internal conflicts, Freud developed a new method of healing.

This method of treatment, still valid today, is linked to the person acting as the therapist and becomes effective as the relationship to the therapist evolves. It is primarily the transfer of feelings and emotions onto the therapist that gradually enables the patient to understand his or her own inner world. This process is called "transference." A number of studies have recently underscored the effectiveness of this method. The new field of neurology has also shown that many assumptions of psychoanalysis are correct and can be proven with the modern methods used in neurology. Thus, leading neurologists agree with psychoanalysis on the following:

- Basic functions of mental activity are below the level of consciousness.
- There is a force that seeks to prevent contents of our psyche from becoming conscious.
- Processes that are not conscious function differently from conscious activities.
- Within our psyche, we can find both a reality principle and a pleasure principle.
- Underlying motives for behavior are due to basic drives (life instincts).

In light of this knowledge of the dynamics of unconscious behavior, the goal of psychoanalysis is to provide help and understanding regarding the development and growth in levels of awareness. That this is working can be ascertained by an accompanying reduction of physical and mental symptoms of illness. Even though psychoanalysis was developed to treat symptoms of psychological illness, it still sees and treats the whole person. This treatment of the whole person includes the development of previously inhibited aspects of a patient's psyche. Furthermore, the psyche itself has been shown to be not a real entity on its own but an expression of whatever relationship a person has to his or her inner and outer world.

Is this understanding of psyche applicable only to our Western world, or can it be applied either partly or wholly to other cultures? How do other cultures understand the term *psychological development*? Let us now address this question.

YOGA

Yoga has developed over the past several decades into a kind of special gymnastics as well as a method of alternative self-treatment. In America and in Europe, we can now find an enormous variety of yoga styles, techniques, and special practices. As yoga has become popularized and mainstream, its original purpose has retreated to the background.

What was yoga originally? How did yogis from the original classical Indian tradition understand yoga? The answer lies in the Yogasūtra.

In the classical Indian tradition, the goal of yoga is described as the ability to concentrate on an object completely and without distraction, and to hold this focus (YS I.2). The exercises within yoga are techniques to develop mental and emotional faculties. This tradition is at least as old as our Western calendar.

Yoga is a part of Indian philosophy. In contrast with psychoanalysis, yoga was not developed to treat psychosomatic illness. Rather, its importance was as a part of Indian philosophy, which developed independently of Western thought in the last two thousand years. One of the characteristics of Indian thought is that there has been no conscious separation between religion and natural sciences and between the body and the mind, as in the West. Instead, there are six so-called *darśanas* (next section), meaning six different perspectives, which encompass all of Indian philosophy. Yoga is one *darśana*, one of these six perspectives. Thus it is a complete view of life according to a particular school of thought.

Yoga presents the development of the human spirit and psyche without using Western polarities such as illness/health, body/mind, subject/object, and so forth. In its practical application, yoga presents methods and means that promote and develop physical as well as mental well-being. Yoga is therefore both a philosophical system and a systematic and structured set of tools to aid development of the whole multifaceted person. The cultural background for this rests clearly within Indian philosophy.

Yoga assumes an underlying dualistic system of pure consciousness (*puruṣa*) and an all-encompassing physical world of matter (*prakṛti*). Consciousness has an eternal, unmeasurable aspect. It is a real and present force and has effects on the world. It has no measurable qualities and is not to be confused with our concept of mind. The closest thing we can compare it to is light. Matter, on the other hand, has three main qualities: movement/energy, heaviness/stasis, lightness/space. These three qualities are linked to three colors: red (movement), black (heaviness), and white (light and space). In Sanskrit, the ancient language of Indian philosophy, these basic forces of life and matter (called *guṇas*) are named *rajas*, *tamas*, and *sattva*. Anything that does not belong to the field of pure consciousness is seen as part of matter. From this perspective, the psyche and its mental contents, as understood from a Western perspective, are all seen as part of the material world!

Matter is in a state of constant movement and transformation within the three qualities just named. This continuous change is called *pariṇāma* in Indian philosophy, and it occurs in the outer world as well as in the inner world of thoughts and feelings.

Amid this continual change, however, there is a fixed and constant point. This is pure consciousness. This consciousness, *puruṣa*, is the central core of a human being. According to yoga philosophy, illness and suffering arise when you confuse your thoughts and ideas, both within the sphere of the material world, with consciousness (your true self). The techniques of yoga are intended to help you to overcome identification with the material and mental world that surrounds you and instead to connect to the real core of your being: pure consciousness.

Yoga discusses these relationships, describes the difficulties on the path to a state of liberation, and offers means and techniques to help find access to this pure consciousness.

Yoga is thus a method to reach pure consciousness, which releases individuals from entangled, constricting identifications, and find true inner freedom. Since both the body and the psyche are part of the material world, there is neither a separation nor a preference between body and psyche. The physical postures are based on techniques that help one get closer to perceiving this state of consciousness. Other techniques include breathing exercises, concentration, meditation, dream analysis, and a meaningful, coherent, everyday lifestyle.

Yoga philosophy and the techniques involved in its practice are contained in concise form in Patañjali's Yogasūtra. This two-thousand-year-old text has been commented on and interpreted many times. However, it is not accessible and cannot be understood without actual practice and concrete explanations from a teacher. The quality of this teaching depends on the authenticity of the teacher and the teacher's own connection to yoga and to his or her own teachers.

Liberation from destructive and limiting identifications via a yoga practice is possible only if the practitioner is in a stable environment, meaning that he or she is physically and mentally healthy. According to yoga, mental suffering and physical illness are the greatest obstructions to freedom. Therefore, yoga first leads to the development of mental and physical stability, which we could call good health. Yoga does not stop here, however, but continues toward the goal of freedom from all possible constrictions.

YOGA AND PSYCHOANALYSIS

Yoga and psychoanalysis can be seen as two completely different systems and means of developing the human psyche: yoga aims to overcome suffering in order to gain spiritual freedom, psychoanalysis to enable people to relinquish suppressed and denied patterns of behavior so that they can better and more easily cope with their lives. Yoga maintains that the nature of a human being is pure consciousness. Psychoanalysis assumes that most mental and psychological processes are unconscious, and that consciousness itself plays a very small part in our human decisions. Psychoanalysis tries to help people to repair their ability to enter into relationships. The goal of yoga is to help people achieve inner freedom. This pertains to personal relationships as well. The goal of psychoanalysis is to help free patients from psychological symptoms that impede their life and thus to help them enjoy their life and function better. The result of psychoanalytic work is a state of inner freedom and mental health. This is the basis, however, for the development provided by yoga. Does yoga, then, start where psychoanalysis leaves off?

Often, we (T.K.V. Desikachar and Hellfried Krusche) have noticed that a yoga student who starts psychoanalysis benefits from this in his or her yoga practice. On the other hand, there are increasing numbers of therapists and psychoanalysts who are also interested in the body and, beyond that, in yoga in general.

We can therefore once again look at the relationship between these two worldviews, both of which seek to change and develop the human psyche. Both systems, yoga and psychoanalysis, offer holistic methods to support human development, even though they were developed in completely different cultural settings. Furthermore, practical experience has shown that the effectiveness of yoga and psychoanalysis, when used together, can be considerably amplified.

The following discussions between a psychoanalyst and a yoga master are intended to represent an authentic interpretation of yoga, as presented in concentrated form in the text of the Yogasūtra, and of psychoanalysis, according to its historical development and its currently practiced form. We have sought to explore whether there are commonalities between yoga and psychoanalysis. If so, these could point to underlying truths in therapeutic approaches and in methods of supporting transformation that are independent of cultural settings and thus universally valid.

There are many different schools of yoga as well as numerous commentaries on the Yogasūtra. Psychoanalysis is also present worldwide in many different applications. Therefore, in order to enable a certain level of verification and comparison, we fixed a methodological approach to limit our discussions to the first nine to eleven sutras of each chapter of the Yogasūtra. We based our interpretation of the text on the teachings and the perspective of T.K.V. Desikachar, who, with his own practice of yoga and the teachings he received from his father on this text over the course of almost three decades, represents an authentic source. This tradition of yoga, which comes from the south of India, is a point of reference for yoga practitioners worldwide. Many schools of yoga have been greatly influenced by T. Krishnamacharya, T.K.V. Desikachar's teacher, and world-famous yoga teachers such as B.K.S. Iyengar, Pattabhi Jois, and Indra Devi, who were also students of T. Krishnamacharya.

We have limited our perspective of psychoanalysis to the schools that base their teachings on Sigmund Freud as taught worldwide by the International Psychoanalytical Association.

In the following text, an open dialogue takes place between yoga and aspects of psychoanalysis to discuss Patañjali's Yogasūtra according to the interpretation by T.K.V. Desikachar. We employ examples and anecdotes to illustrate the different systems, and we will be looking for patterns of similarities as well as differences in each approach.

Our main questions focus on whether human transformation is even possible within culturally constructed systems such as yoga or psychoanalysis, which methods each system applies to support such transformation, and, if change does occur, what such change or transformation might look like.

Conclusions out of this dialogue can then be applied to better understand the general relevance and application of psychoanalysis on the one hand and yoga on the other hand, in both East and West.

At the end, we will explore whether these two important systems, both designed to aid human development, can be used in support and extension of each other. We see this discussion as an important part of the current worldwide dialogue where East and West seek to better understand each other.

ORGANIZATION OF THE BOOK

We will first explain further important background information on yoga and psychoanalysis. After that, the main topic of the book centers on an ongoing discussion of Patañjali's Yogasūtra.

In our first chapter, we will discuss the first eleven sutras of the Yogasūtra chapter 1 and what they tell us about the foundation for psychological development.

In our second chapter, we will discuss the first nine sutras of the Yogasūtra chapter 2 with a view toward answering the question of how methods of treatment are applied to address mental change.

We will address aspects of the results of psychological treatment from both yoga practice and psychoanalysis by looking at the first ten sutras of the Yogasūtra chapter 3.

Then, in the first eleven sutras of the Yogasūtra chapter 4, we will address the question of foundation for transformational change.

Finally, we will look at various aspects of our discussion in light of current societal trends and briefly discuss the implications we see here.

The Dialogue

YOGA AND THE YOGASŪTRA

T.K.V. Desikachar: Let me first introduce you to the Yogasūtra, which is a very special text. The word *sūtra* literally means "to indicate." Let us take the analogy of a set of beautiful pearls, which have to be strung together into a necklace. The sutra is comparable to the string, as it links together a set of invaluable thoughts. The order in which the thoughts are strung together is equally important.

To give you an idea of this, I would also like to briefly describe some of the main qualities of the Yogasūtra. This will be easiest if we also consider the original language in which the sutras were written: Sanskrit.

Let us expand on the special qualities of the Yogasūtra in Sanskrit. They are as follows:

1. *alpākṣaram*: As few words and letters as possible are used.
2. *asandigdham*: There is clear meaning; no ambiguity.
3. *sāravat*: They are full of "juice"; the more you meditate on the meaning, the more you will find.

4. *viśvatomukham*: They contain universal messages that are not intended merely for an individual or specific context.
5. *astobham*: The text is not speculation; it is based on true experiences that human beings can directly encounter.
6. *anavadyam*: The Yogasūtra is full of dignity.

THE VEDAS

The Vedas, our ancient texts passed on from generation to generation, are the source of Indian philosophy, rituals, and values. The Vedas are like an ocean where we can find many different things, depending on our orientation and perspective. Where one person might want to take only salt from the ocean, the next person might take fish, and a third person might just want to use some of the water. Similarly, the Vedas address people in different ways depending on their individual needs and interests.

There are six schools of Vedic philosophy: Mīmāṁsā, Nyāya, Vaiśeṣika, Sāṅkhya, Yoga, and Vedānta. These are called the *vaidika darśana* because they originate from the Vedas. We must be careful not to confuse the Vedas with Hinduism. The Vedas are broader; the focus in Hinduism on God and religion is only one aspect within the more extensive Vedas. Vedānta, which is Hindu philosophy, focuses on God. Mīmāṁsā focuses on ritual. Each of these schools expounds different messages. Yoga focuses on the mind. The sutras are brief, and at the same time they have enormous depth.

YOGA

Meaning within the Yogasūtra is condensed. As we have already discussed, the text itself is concise, dense, deep, and multifaceted. The origins of the Yogasūtra are attributed to a very interesting figure named Patañjali. We know very little about this person, and in fact the origins of important Indian texts are very often surrounded in mystery. Patañjali is frequently described as being half human and half mythical snake, certainly for symbolic reasons. We assume that Patañjali was a rishi, or seer, who had a vision of the greatest truth.

Whenever we start the study of the Yogasūtra, it is our convention to acknowledge and pay respect to the source. Patañjali gave humanity three precious gifts:

1. To better communicate, he gave us Sanskrit grammar.
2. To help us be healthy, he is the source of the Indian medicinal system, Āyurveda.
3. To enable us with a good, clear, strong, and useful mind, he gave humanity yoga, presented within the Yogasūtra.

In our tradition, the Yogasūtra is taught in a particular way. After a year or two of practical instruction in body postures, called *āsanas*, the Yogasūtra would also be included. The teacher would first recite the sutra twice, then we students had to recite the sutra and repeat it three times until we had memorized it, then the teacher would explain the simple meaning. Slowly, during serious study of the Yogasūtra, there would be more stringent instruction, and we would go deeper into the meaning. I had the great fortune of having been taught by my father. In this way, I studied the Yogasūtra with my father nine times. The first lesson was in 1962, the last began in 1985. So for twenty years I studied this text with my father.

I was encouraged to teach the Yogasūtra and began teaching in 1966. The first person I taught was a European. Teaching always raises questions, and my experience was no different. My student was from the West, and my teacher (my father) was from the East. My teacher taught in Sanskrit, and I had to teach in English. As I communicated with my student, occasionally questions arose and I went to my father for clarifications. The Western outlook is different from the Eastern. Some questions Westerners ask, Indians would not. So it became a process of teaching and learning and teaching and learning for me. This interaction with East and West has been a continuing process for me, while at the same time I have remained in touch with my source. For the insight that I have gained into the Yogasūtra, I have to acknowledge both my teacher and my students.

Hellfried Krusche: Now I would like to present the perspective from which I see this dialogue and the viewpoint from which I will pose questions. To do this, I will need to give a brief description of psychoanalysis and of concrete psychoanalytic experience.

Psychoanalysis is an approach within psychotherapy to treat people suffering from unresolved inner conflict. Let's take the example of a successful businessman who still feels like a little child when with his own mother. Although he is not consciously aware of this, he would in fact also like to be taken care of by her in this way. So on the one hand, in a professional context he is a highly successful, independent adult, but on the other hand, he is like a child, highly dependent on his mother. He cannot endure a single day without visiting her. At the same time, he feels that she controls him and does not allow him his freedom. Without realizing it, he is stuck in a deep inner conflict.

Oscillating like this between dependence and autonomy can result in physical symptoms of illness. The cause of such an illness would in this case be inner emotional conflict. The psychoanalytic treatment would be to address this unsolved conflict.

Ordinarily, neither physical treatment nor medication is part of psychoanalysis. "Healing" within psychoanalysis is instead much more a function of "using words"; to do this, a stable and open relationship between the patient and the psychoanalyst must be established. This means that the psychoanalyst must try to win the patient's confidence in order to discuss the patient's underlying basic conflicts within an atmosphere of trust and acceptance. Only then can the analyst bring previously unconscious connections to light and ascertain their significance. In small steps and with the analyst's support, the patient learns to become aware of his or her unconscious conflicts and fears and can then in turn better cope with them in future. This normally leads to a significant reduction of inner tension as well as a greater level of self-awareness and more personal freedom.

Looking again at the example of the businessman, he could then in future determine when he really wants to visit his mother and how far he would like to pursue his desire for more independence. These gains in inner freedom are usually accompanied by a noticeable reduction of both physical symptoms and emotional suffering.

Because of its ability to reduce and at times even eliminate physical symptoms and severe emotional suffering, psychoanalysis is used in many countries as a primarily medical approach within the system of traditional medicine. At the same time, the actual roots of psychoanalysis can be found both in philosophy and in medicine.

Sigmund Freud, who studied and worked in Vienna from 1874 until 1938, is regarded as the founder of psychoanalysis. He was a successful researcher in the field of neurology. He was also very interested in philosophy, and the philosophical ideas of the time certainly influenced his thinking as a researcher in the field of unconscious emotional states.

Freud is credited with developing a theory about and practical approach to treating patients who suffered from so-called hysteria. This approach involved using only words within a properly developed doctor-patient relationship. In developing this theory, he also drew upon his knowledge of Western philosophy. Some of the philosophers who influenced him had themselves been influenced by Indian philosophy. Arthur Schopenhauer was clearly influenced by the Upaniṣads. The German philosopher Paul Deussen, a friend of Friedrich Nietzsche's, was a well-known scholar of Indian philosophy who had translated sutras on Vedānta into German. He saw a connection between the philosophy of ancient Greece and that of the Upaniṣads. These observations point out the possibility of either direct or indirect connections between the philosophical roots of psychoanalysis and Patañjali's Yogasūtra. However, this will not be explored further here.

Although influenced in some capacity by philosophy, Freud placed great importance on the scientific basis of psychoanalysis. Freud was also skeptical of philosophy. He thus tried to steer psychoanalysis according to scientific principles. He founded a scientific society that met to openly discuss ongoing cases; he encouraged psychoanalytic research and published his own articles in scientific journals. For a number of years now there has been a growing amount of psychoanalytic research focused in a systematic way on the treatment success of its therapies.

So how does one become a psychoanalyst? The first step is to complete a degree in either medicine or psychology before starting a training course in psychoanalysis. Training then partly encompasses theory, with even more focus in the practical arena. This means that one must undergo psychoanalytic treatment before subsequently being able to treat others. After Freud's death, his students around the world developed a series of rules and standards according to which one can today practice and teach psychoanalysis. From the very beginning, psychoanalysis has tried to deliver a level of transparency when presenting its treatments and theories. This has enabled it to continue to develop up to the present day. In fact, today there are a number of different theories that are based on psychoanalysis. The common framework remains rooted in Freud's theories on the unconscious and on unconscious conflict as a central cornerstone of the human psyche, as well as on his doctor-patient relationship as an essential element of treatment. The basis of the psychoanalyst's scientific debate remains the analysis of concrete treatment examples deriving from their psychoanalysis.

Part of my training to become a psychoanalyst was a seven-year period during which I went regularly five days a week to my analyst, and I treated my own patients only under the supervision of three additional analysts. Theory was second to practical training and experience. As you can see, this is a rigorous discipline with a primarily practical orientation that is organized and directed by the international community of psychoanalysts.

Psychoanalysts try to see each and every person as a unique individual. To get to know someone, one needs time. Normally we work with our patients over a longer period of time. In this capacity, our work has striking similarities to the serious practice of teaching yoga. But there are differences in the traditions. We try to discuss, present, and evolve our practices and results through scientific discussions.

A further difference is that psychoanalysis is limited to removing inner tension and conflicts. After solving these problems, treatment, and hence the relationship between doctor and patient, ends.

We have agreed to discuss the first nine to eleven sutras of each chapter of the Yogasūtra as a means of introducing each of the four chapters of the text. The discussion from the perspective of psychoanalysis might help interpret the Yogasūtra more clearly for a Western audience. At the same time, we would like to see how relevant psychoanalysis can be for the world of yoga. Perhaps we will thus be able to discover insights that go beyond each of our cultural limitations and can therefore have meaning that transcends individual cultural limitations.

1

What Do Yoga and Relationship Have in Common?

YOGASŪTRA, CHAPTER ONE (*samādhi-pādaḥ*)

T.K.V. Desikachar: After this introduction, I would like to start with the first sutra of the first chapter of the Yogasūtra:

atha yogānuśāsanam
Here begins the authoritative instruction on yoga. (YS I.1)

This sentence can have different meanings, depending on your perspective. When the teacher recites this, it means "Now I am going to share with you the yoga that I have the experience of."

When the student says this, it means "I am committed to you, whatever instruction you may give, I will follow until I experience yoga."

So the same words have two different meanings. While the teacher says, "I have experience; I am able to teach you," the student says, "I am committed to a relationship with you; I am therefore willing to follow your instructions."

The word *committed* is very important. It is the student's promise that he or she is not there for casual study. The student is totally committed, and the teacher expresses satisfaction with that sincerity. In India, teaching something as precious as yoga is never done casually.

For example, when I was just twenty-three years old, my father asked me to come very early for class. It was not easy. But this was the way he tested me. Ancient people had their own unique system to test the student's commitment. When the student approached them the first time, they would give many pretexts not to start. "Come in six months," they would say, or, "We will start the class in January." "We have to wait a month before starting." This is the way the teacher used to test the student's perseverance.

So the message of the first sutra is: The teacher has had the personal experience that gives him or her the authority to teach. Moreover, the teacher is convinced that the student is sincere. From the student's point of view, there is clarity: "I will study yoga, I will stay with this teacher until the teacher teaches me everything."

Hellfried Krusche: The framework of this is very deep commitment and the ability of a student to develop a relationship to the teacher and to yoga. There should not be any doubt or ambivalence regarding this relationship. There should be a serious connection, which may have far-reaching consequences throughout the rest of the student's life. This is difficult for us to understand in the Western world; in fact, many would see it as an unreasonable expectation. However, scientific research has shown that a connection and identification with a therapist, for example with a psychoanalyst, can be very conducive to the transformative process. We see this again and again in psychoanalysis. It is clear for us psychoanalysts that it is crucial for us to experience long-lasting relationships. Only through the experience of such a relationship can we actually know what change really is. Part of this experience is realizing that negative feelings also have their place within a relationship. Only when we have learned how to constructively use negative feelings within a relationship are we capable of dealing with that which we encounter in the relationship with our patients in a skillful and helpful way. This is why, in Western psychoanalysis, therapists first have to go through a longer period of therapy before being ready to take on patients themselves. They have to be able to understand their patients on an emotional as well as an intellectual level. So you see, there are similarities between our cultures.

The most important thing for the therapist is to develop the capacity to be open with his or her patient and to interact without prejudice or having any preconceived notions. A good therapist who is able to do this from the start can be receptive to messages from the patient from the very first meeting. When therapist and patient meet for the first time in this way, there should be something like what you described. This capacity to be open and start a new relationship is thus similar to what you describe with yoga.

But there is an important difference. What you deem essential at the beginning of yoga teaching, we see as something that has to be developed over a long period—it may even be the final result of therapy. It seldom exists straight from the outset.

D: Perhaps the difference is not really so great. As I said, what my father first taught me was simple and superficial. He went step by step. This is for two reasons. First, the student has to understand. The teacher needs to ensure this. Second, the interest to learn or experience cannot be imposed. As the student experiences more and more in practice, the teacher unfolds more and more meaning. It is a process. That is why the word *anu*, meaning "to follow," is used. The less the student follows, the less he or she experiences, and vice versa. Yoga is not merely intellectual. It is about inner transformation. And as we will see as we go on, yoga is also relationship.

H: Do you mean that transformation happens through relationship?

D: Yes. For example, the first thought that came into my mind while starting this work was that I had to acknowledge Patañjali.

Then I wanted to acknowledge my teacher, my father. This is relationship.

Coming back to the first sutra, *atha yogānuśāsanam* is about experience. Let me contrast this with the first sutra in Hinduism, called the Brahmasūtra. It says: *athāto brahma-jijñāsā*. "Let us inquire into Brahman." This is intellectual, while *atha yogānuśāsanam* is experiential.

Let me put this in context for you. In the beginning, when I started my yoga lessons I told my father that I did not believe in God. He said, "If you don't believe in God, that is fine." Then in 1964 we came to the sutra about *Īśvara-praṇidhāna*, which means that you recognize and trust in a higher power. He said, "This is not important for you. Let us go to the next sutra." In 1984, when I asked him to teach the Yogasūtra based on his own experience, he said, "The basic experience I have of yoga is: total faith in God! For me, total faith in God is the only way to change a state of mind."

So, to repeat, in the beginning my teacher was very flexible. He worked according to the inner needs of his student. As the relationship grew stronger, he began to speak of his own experience and authority. This is very important because yoga is neutral. We mistake yoga for Hinduism. Yoga is not Hinduism. My father had great faith, but he never imposed his beliefs on me.

H: You said yoga has to be taught step-by-step. It seems like the teacher tries to reach the student at his or her level, and the student tries to do the same with the teacher. So the student follows the teacher, and at the same time the teacher follows the student. From the very beginning, each side moves toward the other to build a relationship. And this relationship should allow openness and trust to develop. Is that correct?

D: Yes!

H: So this relationship between teacher and student should strive for openness and commitment?

D: Absolutely.

H: So trust (called *śraddhā* in Sanskrit), and the capacity of one being in touch with the other, should be developed during this process at the deepest level possible. Any obstacle should be removed?

D: Yes. That is why in Sanskrit the words used are not *atha yoga śāsanam* but rather *atha yogānuśāsanam. Śāsanam* is a command and means something that must be followed and practiced. However, *anuśāsanam* indicates respect for the person since *anu* means "to follow"; *anuśāsanam* is therefore something that can be followed and practiced.

H: This is a process taking place?

D: Yes, it is a dynamic process and not an order. That is why the word *anu* is so important. The person who has the experience and the person who wants to have it must both come into contact with each other. It is a living relationship, not a sheet of paper. I would like to clarify something before continuing. The relationship that we are talking about is focused only on yoga. For instance, my relationship with a politician I am teaching is not about politics, but only about yoga. This is very clearly stated in the Upaniṣads. We have to respect the person; there is no other kind of relationship. You may recall that a few years ago you mentioned that you did not go to the concert of one of your patients. You distanced yourself in order to protect the therapeutic relationship. This is not always easy. There should be discipline on the part of the yoga teacher. We should not go too deeply into the everyday life of our students. The yoga teacher must be disciplined and practice self-restraint. As I said, it is not easy, but if I treat someone as a powerful politician, then I will not have the authority of a teacher. And the student will not respect me. That is why the words *atha yogānuśāsanam* are so important. Our relationship is about transformation of the mind and the psyche and nothing else!

H: If you give advice, it should be understood only in terms of yoga and transformation.

D: Yes. This is why *atha* is a very important and powerful word. *Atha* also means "attention, reference, commitment, and awareness of what is to be done." I repeat, *atha* is a very strong word. My father would insist on our reciting the first sutra after every sutra:

atha yogānuśāsanam
yogaś citta-vṛtti-nirodhaḥ
atha yogānuśāsanam
tadā draṣṭuḥ svarūpe'vasthānam
atha yogānuśāsanam
vṛtti-sārūpyamitaratra

H: So when you are in contact with your students, how do you make the distinction between yoga-related issues and normal life situations?

D: A friend of mine likes wine. When he comes here, I always get him a very good wine. It is for him to decide whether he will drink the wine or not. The second thing is, in ancient times the young student would stay with a teacher for eight years. Today it is not like that. Some of my students are older than me. It is a different situation. And transformation too is different.

We have to be clear about *dharma*. I do not like to interfere. Many of my students ask me, What can I do for you? I say, I only want the connection with you. This ethical framework is very important. I interact with my students only as a yoga teacher. My father taught the king of Mysore, but he never accepted any kind of gift from him. The king sometimes sent him jewelry, but my father wouldn't even touch it. He sent it back immediately. Authority is lost when the student becomes the authority because of this kind of power.

H: From the beginning you demand a lot from your yoga students. The requirements in the West for psychotherapy patients are not the same as this. In our setup, patients have to come, respect the setting, pay the fees, and speak freely about that which preoccupies them. Initially, there is also a process on a superficial level. This should be maintained for a period of time to protect the young and developing relationship.

So in fact, when it comes to the qualities of the relationship, there is a similarity with yoga. Many analysts today agree that if you are able to undertake and build a very deep and long-lasting relationship, nearly every mental illness can be overcome, even the results of severe mental trauma. The hurdle is that many patients, when they enter psychotherapy, fear loss of control. So they try to undermine the developing relationship in order to protect themselves. They want this relationship, but at the same time they resist it. This interferes and tends to destroy the relationship. How to deal with this is one of the main problems in psychotherapy—how to sustain a relationship, how to protect it and go along with it. How do you deal with this problem of establishing a relationship in yoga? How do you protect and develop it?

D: Building a relationship is difficult. It takes time to build confidence and trust. This is not easy. In India, there is a saying: Only four ears must hear—teacher and student. That is why in transformation there is only one connection: teacher-student, one to one. They say in Sanskrit, if you want to learn something that will help you transform, it is like surgery. One doctor cannot operate on several people at the same time. This setting and ambience should be confidential. Not only should it *be* confidential, it should *appear* confidential. Like when I closed the door for our session. Only you and I are here. The resistance to such a close relationship is often enormous. There are lots of problems, like possible shame and questions of trust. Not everyone who has gone through yoga has been transformed.

Today there are also too many choices. In ancient times there was only one teacher. As we say, many people are "collectors" but not "connectors." That is why many people have not truly benefited from yoga. So in both the West and the East, we have similar problems.

Also, there is fear. Fear of making a mistake, fear of disappointing, fear of being exploited. That is why the connection between student and teacher is confined to yoga only. Even gender is not important. For example, when Patañjali taught yoga, the students did not even see his face. There was a curtain between them. So the student only heard the teacher's instruction. What is the symbolism here? It is that the teacher-student connection is not physical but spiritual. Patañjali said, "Nobody should open the curtain. Otherwise he will burn to ashes." There are two sides—the teacher has to earn trust, the student has to apply effort.

Proper compensation is another topic. In our tradition, the teacher asks the student for fees at the end of the teaching. The teacher will decide the fees depending on the transformation and the resources of the student, based on his or her probable future. And the student, if he or she trusts the teacher, will never disappoint him. So, for example, after seventeen years of teaching, the teacher may say, "Now you have developed and transformed, you can go to the next stage of life and this is what I want you to pay." It may be a cow or it may be gold. At the end of this period of teaching, the teacher also gives these instructions:

1. Tell the truth!
2. Follow your *dharma*, your correct path in life!
3. Do not assume that you have completed your studies!
4. Continue your self-inquiry (*svādhyāya*).
5. Now pay the fees, start a family, and have children.

What I want to clarify is that the teacher does not want slavery. The teacher wants to serve the student. When the student has been transformed and has become a wiser person, only then does the teacher expect something. If the student has not changed, the teacher will not feel comfortable.

For a teacher, the student is very important, because the transmission of what the teacher got from his or her own teacher will die if there is no student. The river will cease to flow. When he was ninety-nine years old, my father would tell me: "Don't miss your classes, because when I die all that I received from my teacher and haven't passed on will die." There was the feeling that one is obliged to transmit what one has received to the next generation. Otherwise you do not show your gratitude to your teacher. The happiest moment for the teacher is when the student is better than the teacher, when the student shows greater mastery at any level.

H: Like a relationship between father and child.

D: Exactly! There is a quote: "I want to be surpassed by no one apart from my own child."

H: In our society, there are only a very few examples of this kind of personal passing on of what one has learned. We see it, for example, in the education of artists, painters, musicians. We also find it within the sphere of training psychoanalysts in the analytic process, which is the practical part of a psychoanalyst's education. Here, students training to become psychoanalysts undergo analysis of their personal experiences for several years. After this, they can become analysts themselves and might even work with their teachers. I work with my teacher now. It is a great honor and a pleasure. There may be a situation where a student even becomes better than his or her teacher. This is not intended, but it may happen.

So in this process, there is a development within a relationship that is comparable to the process of yoga. The difference in this training in the West, however, is that it is institutionalized and maintained by various authorities. There is also a scientific community that monitors the process. There is a limited exposure to the public world, and there are set standards and expectations that must be met. Is this comparable to yoga?

D: You know, we cannot dictate to our students. The most essential process happens in the heart of the student. Therefore they should be open. This is demonstrated in the Bhagavad Gītā. In this text, Lord Krishna interacts openly with Arjuna and explains the need to act honestly and in accordance with one's *dharma*. In the end, Arjuna is convinced that he should indeed take action.

Today, more than ever, we cannot command. Respect must be earned and not demanded. The two conditions are authority and love. Authority stems from competence, while love comes from a long relationship, friendship, care, attention, and respect. Many students have left their yoga teachers because the latter aspect was neglected.

D: Let us move to the second sutra:

yogaś citta-vṛtti-nirodhaḥ

This sutra defines yoga clearly. There are three very important words: *citta vṛtti nirodhaḥ.* The word *citta* in Sanskrit means "something that is very close to consciousness," but it is not consciousness itself. Left to itself, it dominates. *Citta* comes from the word *cit*, which means "consciousness." *Citta* means "that which is so close to consciousness that it is almost consciousness." In Sanskrit we say, "That consciousness which pretends to be consciousness is *citta*."

Vṛtti comes from a Sanskrit word meaning "interaction"—for example, like a trader who sells something and receives something. This interaction is possible only because of the connection. Otherwise there is no interaction. So it means one thing moves to another.

Nirodha means here that all these interactions are decided by consciousness, and only consciousness determines the interaction.

I want to look at a flower. I want to meditate on this flower. If my consciousness is very strong, then my mind will not wander elsewhere. I want to see the flower. "What is this flower? Have I ever offered it to somebody?" All my consciousness is on the flower. When *citta*, which can function in so many ways in so many fields, is confined to a particular focus by the power of consciousness, nothing else will enter this field. So attention is concentrated totally on what has been chosen and nothing else. This is called "the state of yoga." Obviously this cannot happen if consciousness is weak and *citta*, which pretends to be consciousness, is very strong.

Later sutras talk about the five different actions of *citta*:

- correct perception (*pramāṇa*)
- incorrect perception (*viparyaya*)
- imagination (*vikalpa*)
- complete suspension of mental activities, called deep sleep (*nidrā*)
- memory (*smṛti*)

Now, perception can be many things. It can be the flower in front of me, and the next moment it can be that I want to make a phone call. Memory is also infinite. We don't know how many memories there are. Imagination too is countless. So the field of the *citta* is infinite. The aim of yoga is to choose one thing from this infinite variety and to stay with the chosen focus for a length of time. Let me try to put this idea more simply. This sutra means that we need to focus, and to focus we need a goal. Then, we simply focus on what is in front of us and nothing else.

If I am engaged in the past, I cannot see what is in front of me now. That is why I say: I have to be present in the present. I am not with you, Hellfried, whom I met at eight o'clock; I am not with my wife, whom I saw after that; I should not be with another student, whom I met later. This means that I have to cut certain things out of my memory and imagination. *Citta-vṛtti-nirodhaḥ* means "to disconnect from anything other than what is in front of me."

The focus could be the body, it could be breath, or it could be an idea. At this moment, my focus is to present to you the Yogasūtra based on what I have learned from my father and my experience in a way that is consistent with our project of seeking common ground between Freud and Patañjali.

Focusing on the body is called *āsana*, focusing on the breath is called *prāṇāyāma*. For *āsana*, we need some tools like breath, movements, observation, and focus on certain parts of the body. To quote my father, yoga also consists of *pratyāhāra*, which is to withdraw the senses from an exterior, worldly focus, and *dhyāna*, which is meditation.

To give an example: I used the following method to teach an eighteen-year-old girl from the United States. I told her that I wanted her to start with the breath, first breath and then body. Only when the movement of the body is over should the breath end. So if the breath is eight seconds, the movement must be only six seconds. Start with the breath and then go on to the body movement, and when the latter is over, you continue for two seconds. That is how I introduced yoga to her. It was not easy for her. Initially the breath was five seconds, then it was eight seconds, and so on. In this way, she experienced yoga. So to summarize, *āsana* begins when we focus on the body.

H: This reminds me of what we call the relationship between consciousness and preconsciousness in psychoanalysis. Freud describes consciousness as the light of a lamp. At the center of this light lies our consciousness. Surrounding this light, however, most of what we live, feel, and remember is preconscious in that we are not focused on it. That which is not within the center of our conscious attention is called "preconsciousness." Preconscious knowledge and thoughts accompany us constantly in our daily life, without our being aware of it.

For example, when we drive a car we are aware of only a fraction of the actions we perform. These preconscious activities have an influence on our conscious thoughts and behavior; they impact our actions and our thinking in such a way that we do not even notice it. Most of our fantasies are preconscious.

When we practice psychoanalysis, the aim is to allow part of preconsciousness to emerge into consciousness. We invite our patients to speak freely, and we try to establish connections between unconscious and conscious thoughts. As this happens, little by little, preconscious and unconscious thoughts lose their influence on overall behavior. Hidden desires come into the conscious arena and thus lose their power. This is so effective because the preconscious has a close connection to the deep, underlying unconscious. Our method is thus to reach the unconscious via the preconscious. The unconscious has patterns that influence our behavior and of which we cannot become aware without accessing the preconscious.

We are therefore trying to strengthen and extend consciousness. But we do this by bringing preconsciousness into consciousness. Freud used the sentence *Where id was, ego shall be*. That which we call consciousness is established by using language. We thus try to extend the field of consciousness and become aware of unconscious intentions by inviting sub- and preconscious thoughts into the arena of conscious analysis. Your emphasis on the special attention of a teacher for his or her student is therefore not a foreign concept to us in psychoanalysis. One of the leading theorists, Wilfred Bion, pointed to the importance of remaining inwardly open and receptive to our patients. He expressed this in the famous phrase *no memory, no desire*. This means that in each session the psychoanalyst should endeavor to see his or her patient in a fresh light, as if seeing the person again for the very first time. It is just as you said earlier: you were seeing me not as the Hellfried from eight o'clock in the morning, but as the Hellfried I am at four o'clock in the afternoon.

I am astounded that despite the different cultures and traditions of our two systems, there are nonetheless so many important similarities regarding our approaches to interacting.

But there is also a marked difference. For us in the West, the concept of becoming one with something in the way you have described is difficult for us truly to achieve. For instance, when I observe myself, there are nearly always different thoughts occurring at the same time. There have been only a very few occasions in my life when I have felt something like the unity between focus and perception that you have described.

Could we say that your definition of yoga is something for us to strive for? For normal people without special training, there will typically be very few occasions, if any, when they experience complete unity with and focus on what they are doing. Perhaps yoga in this context has an important lesson for us in the West?

Apart from this difference, the overall direction of yoga and psychoanalysis appears similar. In yoga, you strengthen consciousness by practicing appropriate exercises. In psychoanalysis, we use language to try to make the unconscious conscious by going through the preconscious. We both use the vehicle of relationship to accomplish this.

D: There is a reason Patañjali chose the word *citta*. There are two Sanskrit words for the mind. One is *manas* and the other *citta*. *Manas* is related to the mind's structure but is very close to the senses. *Citta* is the same mind, but it is not close to the senses. It is closer to consciousness. If I am very agitated or disturbed, *citta* becomes *manas*. When I am a little more attentive, *manas* becomes *citta*. So the quality of the mind shifts.

I will give you an example: I am talking to you now. You were responding, and I was listening. My wife came to see me a little while ago; I could see her through the window. She usually never comes unless it is important. But I made the decision to stay here. This is *citta*. Suppose I was not close to consciousness; I would then have said, "Hellfried, please excuse me, my wife is waiting." So the mind is a fluid thing in yoga. When it is very close to consciousness, consciousness is the master. When it is not, the senses are the masters. It is not possible to stay in a state of yoga when there is an inner state of agitation.

Effort must be put in so that *manas* becomes *citta*. In other words, we must shift the mind from a state dominated by the senses to a state where it is closer to consciousness.

H: This fluctuation of the psyche between two states is something we also observe in psychoanalysis. Here we call this a movement between two inner psychological "positions," where one is seen as an integrating force and the other a disintegrating force. The disintegrating force is called a "paranoid-schizophrenic" position and is a state we can fall into if suffering from extreme fear. In this condition, we are not able to formulate any positive or logically connected thoughts, whereas in an integrated inner position we are able to reflect and understand.

D: The second sutra in the first chapter defines the goal of yoga and also defines the ways and means to achieve it.

H: So the goal as you define it is to bring the mental-emotional body closer to consciousness. This involves moving the psyche from a state closely influenced by the senses to one that is closer to consciousness. This requires, however, a level of inner development, which will always involve a certain amount of emotional effort. Is this correct?

D: My father used to say we need a lot of effort for a moment of yogic experience. It is not possible to stay continuously in the state where consciousness is the master for long. But that one moment is worth trying for, because we discover something: a very special joy.

H: Can you describe this? What is it that we experience in this state? Is it the surprise of being in touch with something new? Or is it to see things differently from before? What is it?

D: This is what the next sutra answers:

> *tadā draṣṭuḥ svarūpe'vasthānam*
> Then the ability to understand the object fully and correctly is apparent. (YS I.3)

The result of this yogic experience is the discovery of our own consciousness, the power of this consciousness, the light of this consciousness, and clarity.

H: So it is my own light I see? It is not something supernatural, as many maintain?

D: It is clarity! Sigmund Freud's metaphor of a lamp, which you mentioned earlier, is a beautiful example. First there is darkness, and then there is a lamp. When the lamp starts to burn, two things happen. There is light, and because of the light we see the object in front of us. That is why we say consciousness is what perceives and which helps us to perceive. It sees, it can be seen, and it helps us see correctly.

H: Who sees consciousness? Who is the perceiver of consciousness?

D: Consciousness is the seer of consciousness. It sees itself. This is why it is defined as *draṣṭuḥ*, which means "that which perceives itself and that which helps us to perceive other things." Otherwise, if we said something else is consciousness, who would be able to see it? We will see later that consciousness, which perceives itself, is always aware of the mind. It is the master. It does not change like the mind. It is like the king who knows what is happening in his country.

H: What about spiritual experiences? What about the experiences of God or a higher force, which many meditators and yoga practitioners have spoken about?

D: To be very frank, in the Yogasūtra, when we meditate on God, we never meet God. We discover ourselves.

Refer to sutra 28 in the first chapter. This sutra says that by meditating on God, we will have a vision of our own consciousness, and many obstacles will be overcome. This is what is so different between

Hinduism and yoga. The Yogasūtra doesn't say you will have a vision of God. Because with due respect, God, or *Īśvara*, is a projection of the mind. It is a positive projection. I can see a flower or a mountain, but God? It is a concept. This is extraordinary. Patañjali says that even if you meditate on *Īśvara*, who is God, you won't see God but only your own consciousness. This is why Vedānta is not very happy with yoga. Because in Vedānta the focus is God. Not so in the Yogasūtra. The goal of yoga is to see things truthfully, correctly, and clearly: total clarity of perception. The object of our attention could be the body or it could be the breath. It could also be a life problem. Whatever it is, attention in the present moment is important. So to summarize, yoga is a state of mind where we are totally present. When we are totally present, we have a vision of what is in front of us, and ultimately we have the vision of our self, which is beyond the mind.

That is what the sutra says. When a person is totally focused and is able to stay focused, two things happen:

1. There is total clarity of the perception of the focus.
2. There is also an experience of consciousness.

Consciousness has three qualities:

- It is. This means it is not an illusion, it is real. In Sanskrit this is called *sat*, "it exists."
- It is always awake; in Sanskrit this is called *cit*.
- It has certain qualities that are beyond normal, everyday emotions like sorrow and joy. In Sanskrit this is described as *ānanda*, meaning "without limitation."

Sat-cit-ānanda:

1. It is real.
2. It is always present.
3. It has no suffering, it is unlimited.

Earlier, when I referred to my wife coming here, it was not my mind that decided to stay. The mind presented my wife. I decided for the interaction with you. That "I" is other than the mind. Mind will go to my wife, I will stay with you. That is *cit*.

H: But who decides? Who is this "I"?

D: *Cit* decides. There are two masters: one is the mind (you could also say the intellect), the other is pure consciousness (*cit*, *draṣṭuḥ*, or *puruṣa*). Most often it is the mind that has the upper hand, but sometimes it is this pure consciousness. Because of sentiment or curiosity I could have attended to my wife, but I thought to myself, "The house is not burning." If the mind had been a bit fickle, I would have gone to her. This is a question of priority. This happens only if consciousness is strong.

The fourth sutra says: *vṛtti-sārūpyamitaratra*. In other moments, when we are not in the state of yoga, the mind decides everything. Perception is then that which is presented by the mind and not necessarily that which is true. Our perception could then, for example, be based on imagination or memory. As already mentioned, we have two types of perception: correct and distorted. Distorted perception could be based more on memory or other movements of the mind than on reality. When the mind is agitated, distortion is more likely to occur. When stability returns, the mind helps us see things more clearly. That is why we say the mind is a cruel master, but it is a faithful servant.

H: Surely this requires a certain level of inner balance. For example, is it fair to say that you know your wife very well? If your relationship with your wife were uncertain, you might have reacted differently. Maybe then you would have given in to the temptation to find out what she wanted. We could apply this to other situations.

If the relationships in our lives are harmonious and in balance, we might then be able to come into contact with *cit*. The mind is not independent from the environment around us. The most powerful relationships we have are those with our closest relatives. The same thing is true for our inner world—in other words, the way we interact with the internal pictures we have of people in our internal world. We call these "the internal objects." Both the world of our internal objects and the external world of concrete objects and relationships are important. Our mind or consciousness is not so powerful that it can overcome everything that surrounds us. The inner world and the outer world are both important, and if we do not have internal balance, we cannot make conscious decisions.

D: At 11:00, my work is supposed to be with you. This is called making a choice. If I look at the flower, it is the flower that is at the center of my consciousness. Even if I see a beautiful car, the best car in the world, the choice I can make is the flower, and I can stay with that. That is why the Sanskrit word *nirodha* is used. It is a very strong word. We need to have strength to stay in focus. A weak system cannot do that. There could be distraction from outside or from inside us. So in order to practice this type of concentration, there must be great inner strength.

H: Can we say that this capacity emerged because of a very long period of training with the appropriate exercises? Also, your current environment is well organized. It has become increasingly peaceful, and most of the conflicts from the past have been resolved, not all, but most of them. So one could say that there are not many difficulties from the past or from the environment. Your immediate situation is well balanced. If there were unresolved problems in your internal or external world, might it have been more difficult even for you to remain focused?

D: Absolutely.

H: So if we are to teach people yoga, we have to show them how to bring peace and clarity to their past and to the present. So much depends on our internal and external state of balance. Would you therefore agree that in teaching yoga, we have to work on problems concerning both external relationships and internal issues?

D: Yes.

H: So if someone wants to become free with the help of yoga, he or she must resolve open issues from the past. This is very similar to the approach of psychoanalysis.

D: Yes, that is what the second chapter of the Yogasūtra talks about. Here the issue is how we can prepare so that we have an experience of yoga. We have to clean up the mess in and around us so that pure consciousness can unfold.

This is why pure consciousness is not merely an idea. It is something very strong. It has great strength. This is often not understood. We can compare it to the sun. The sun is very strong. Sometimes there are clouds, but the sun is not destroyed. After some time the clouds disappear, and then we see the sun again. To come back to our sutra once again: *tadā draṣṭuḥ svarūpe'vasthānam*. This says: "In the state of yoga we have the revelation of our own pure consciousness."

tadā—now, at this moment
draṣṭuḥ—pure consciousness
svarūpe'vasthānam—appears

Otherwise, as it is said in the next sutra, we confuse the mind with pure consciousness: *vṛtti-sārūpyamitaratra*.

An important Sanskrit word is used here: *draṣṭuḥ*. That which perceives, that which can see. The mind helps the process, but it does not perceive itself. *Draṣṭuḥ* means "that which can perceive everything," including the mind. Even if I am agitated, pure consciousness, with the help of the mind and the senses, can perceive. For example, "This is Hellfried. He is wearing glasses."

So *draṣṭuḥ* is that which can perceive itself and anything else. In the fourth chapter of the Yogasūtra, the word *cit* is also used to describe this state. The fourth chapter discusses the highest state of yoga, where we have no ambitions and the mind does not fluctuate. *Draṣṭuḥ* is then, in its true nature, beyond distortion. That is the power of pure consciousness. This is the last sutra of the fourth chapter.

What this third sutra in the first chapter means is that when we are in the state of yoga, when we are focused and not agitated, *draṣṭuḥ*, which is in us, can perceive itself, anything outside of us, and anything inside us.

H: What determines whether or not we can experience this kind of perception?

D: When *draṣṭuḥ* is the master, there is no mistake. Perception is correct. When it is not the master, we go by what the mind says based on its projections and on memory. This is true for you and me and anybody else. In an attentive state, *draṣṭuḥ* is the master. That is then yoga.

When there is no attention, *draṣṭuḥ* is virtually dormant. It is not active. This is what the fourth sutra says: *vṛtti-sārūpyamitaratra. Itaratra* means "in other times." It means when there is no attention, the mind presents reality based on x-memories and y-imaginations. At that moment, this is taken as the true and correct perception. The Yogasūtra presents the mind as an instrument, not as a master. However, the instrument often appears as the master. For example, take the modern habit of working on a computer. People have become so accustomed to working with computers that now they sometimes feel they cannot think without one. Is the computer, or the person using the computer, the master? Similarly, the mind is a beautiful instrument, but it is only an instrument, not the real master!

H: Within psychoanalysis, we have a different approach to consciousness. We link consciousness to language. Language in turn regulates relationships. We do not have the methods to work with consciousness as you do in yoga. We see the motor for the activities of the mind and the psyche as located within deeply rooted fears and unconscious conflicts. We analysts try to transform the mind by becoming conscious of these internal problems and conflicts. In this way, we try to let a kind of inner unity arise that can then lead to more internal space to develop one's level of conscious awareness. We are therefore not trying to practice the art of concentrating the mind on one single focus, but instead place great importance on the ability to engage in deep relationships. We make the assumption that the ability to uphold a long-lasting relationship to a specific person helps us to develop certain human strengths. Just think, for example, of the abilities we can experience when we fall in love!

D: For the mind to function, it needs energy. In deep sleep, this appears to be missing. We can imagine that pure consciousness, also called *draṣṭṛ*, is something like the sun. For us, the sun is that which gives light and thus enables us to see. Sunlight is thus something like pure consciousness. We call human energy *prāṇa.* The energy that radiates to any part of the human system is comparable to sunlight. When we are sleeping, the sun appears to be gone, it is dark. But just like the sun, consciousness is not really sleeping. When we get up in the morning, we remember our dreams.

H: How is this possible? Does consciousness transform itself in sleep? How can it be there and at the same time not there at all? According to psychoanalysis, we don't normally truly remember our actual dreams; instead, we remember our interpretation of them upon waking. So we actually remember only that which our mind has already processed and changed. Pure consciousness remains hidden to us. We would say that we only ever see that which has surfaced to a conscious level; to arrive at that point, it goes through a number of transformations. In yoga, how do you understand the difference between a waking and a sleeping state?

D: Consciousness can expand and contract. When I am disturbed and agitated, I cannot sleep. When I am not agitated and when I am peaceful, it is easy to sleep. The sun rises and sets in its own way; it is not affected by external changes. The mind, however, is different. How does an agitated mind prevent pure consciousness from withdrawing, for example, when we have trouble falling asleep? It is a very good question, for which the answer is not clear. If *draṣṭṛ* is the master, how is this possible? How does pure consciousness get connected and how does it get disconnected? Is it the power of our consciousness or something else? We don't know, although there are various theories. In yoga, sleep is a state of mind. In Vedānta, sleep is a state of consciousness. Vedānta describes four types of consciousness:

1. wakefulness
2. deep sleep
3. dream state
4. the highest state of yoga, where we are so absorbed that we have an extraordinary experience, which is total silence

This fourth state is contained in the sound "OM," which is made up of the following:

1. A—waking state
2. U—deep sleep
3. M—dream state
4. silence—highest state

In the Yogasūtra, deep sleep is called *nidrā*, which as I mentioned before is one of the five movements of the mind (of *citta*). This is different from the Upaniṣads. Something happens to the mind where it is almost covered by darkness. This is deep sleep. No movement of the mind takes place and hence no comprehension happens. Clouds completely cover the sun, so there is no light. It is not the sun that changes.

It is the clouds. This is unique to Patañjali, to present sleep as a state of mind and not as a state of pure consciousness.

H: If I can summarize, you are stating that pure consciousness is the constant background of everything. It is only clouded or hidden by the different states of mind. So we have to focus on the mind if we want to get to know pure consciousness?

D: Yes. Yogasūtra chapter 2, sutra 20, says this. Perception happens through the mind. If the mind is colored, perception is colored. If the mind is clear, perception is clear. As a psychoanalyst, how do you explain when a client comes to you and says, "I am very agitated and completely upset"? How do you explain this condition? Does it come from pure consciousness or from somewhere else?

H: From the perspective of psychoanalysis, this agitated state clearly comes from the inner world of the psyche, which then influences the mind and its perception. We assume that there is always a provable cause for this kind of mental agitation. Usually, however, people are not aware of these causes and therefore they do not understand the inner connections. We try to help people become conscious or aware of these inner links. Once they become aware of these influences, they can free themselves of a great deal of mental agitation. Psychoanalysis believes that the manner in which we process internal and external influences determines our emotional states.

Consciousness is for us a neutral quality that can be present or absent. For example, we might be aware of an internal conflict, or we might be unaware of it. We also assume that some unconscious internal conflicts can manifest themselves as tension in the body, pain, or other physical symptoms. The closer a problem or conflict comes to the surface of consciousness, the easier it is to become conscious of this situation and the easier it then becomes for us to solve the conflict. Consciousness itself, however, does not have any quality or energy. This is a key difference between psychoanalysis and yoga. When I want to address a person in an agitated state, the way I would go about it would certainly depend on whether I know the person or not. Let us say I know the person. In this case I would say, "Since I know you, I realize that you have your reasons for being so agitated, but maybe you are not aware of them. Let us try to find them together. What happened to you yesterday, the day before, last week before you came to me, before that, or even while you were driving to me? Let us analyze the situation from the outside and the inside."

I would try to understand what happened to the person and what hurt him or her or caused the conflict. I am sure that some unconscious internal conflict is influencing the situation. Together with the person, we try to find the reason for this. Often we find that some cause for a recent conflict was briefly considered consciously by the person and then rejected, thus again becoming unconscious and getting mixed up with other, deeper internal conflicts. We have to overcome this mechanism of rejection or repression to understand it, make it reappear, and talk about it. As a result, we can increase a person's level of consciousness.

For example, I recently was shopping in the supermarket, and since I was in a hurry, I walked right past a patient of mine without recognizing her. I simply didn't see her. She, on the other hand, saw me and wondered why I didn't stop to greet her. Initially, she did not experience any emotional reaction as a result of this. However, on her way to my practice, she fell into an increasingly bad mood, and she didn't know why. When she arrived, she was confused and silent. Only after we spoke about some of the concrete situations she had experienced over the last few days did the episode in the supermarket occur to her. At first she mentioned this in a roundabout way. I said that perhaps the fact that I didn't see her and hence did not greet her could have insulted her. At this point, she was able to reflect and she realized that indeed this was the event that had caused her recent conflict. Only by talking about it did we realize that this patient has a tendency to overlook anything that might cause her to feel insulted.

She simply shuts out such experiences and forgets them. Afterward, she feels bad and she doesn't know why.

In this case, several things happened:

1. The patient had to think about how she perceives certain things and does not perceive other situations.
2. She realized that I am listening to her. She identified with my attention to her and to the fact that I am taking her seriously. She also thus became more aware of herself.
3. As soon as she realized that I can empathize with her, she became able to address her own feelings. She no longer had to hide from herself.
4. Now we started to work together jointly—my consciousness and her consciousness merged, and together we tried to find relevant connections that she alone would not have been able to find.
5. The point here was to find causes and connections that have led to this behavior. She had been ashamed of being jealous, and she had not dared take these feelings seriously. As a result, she had hidden her emotions from herself, and she had repressed her awareness of the situation. This in turn had led to her feelings of agitation or annoyance and to a sense of being insulted, but not to knowing why or where this came from.
6. Understanding the situation and the dynamics within it led to increased consciousness. Now I could tell the patient why this encounter had caused her to get so upset, and I could help her to become more aware of herself and better understand her own emotions and behavior.

D: By looking at this example, we see that the mind has different states of consciousness. These are presented in the sutras.

The most extremely agitated state, in which we don't know what is happening to us, is called *kṣiptam.* In this state, I am not at all aware of what I am doing. This is the most chaotic state of mind.

The next level is a state where I have no interest in anything. I feel dull. I don't feel like doing anything. This is called *mūḍham.*

The next state is one in which I am a little confused, not very clear. That is perhaps a state where someone would go to an analyst. At least here we have the clarity to ask for help. This is called *vikṣiptam.*

Finally, there is a state in which there is attention. One is not agitated. This is the first state of yoga. It is called *ekāgratā.*

These are the various states of mind.

H: What would you say about people who are perhaps very aware, but who split off a part of their personality? They are very focused, but their feelings are absent.

D: In yoga, pure consciousness is the master. But it is true that there are many old conditionings, or *saṁskāras.* These could, for example, lead to a split in the psyche. This would perhaps be a case for psychoanalysis.

Let us now look at the next sutra:

> *vṛtti-sārūpyamitaratra*
> The ability to understand the object is simply replaced by the mind's conception of that object or by a total lack of comprehension. (YS I.4)

When the mind is not near to *cit,* it is near the senses. Then it is called *manas.* This is the case in the absence of the state of yoga.

When the mind perceives something in this state, it behaves as if the perception is true, but in fact this false perception is based on the mind's own structure and not on reality. It is as if an actor onstage is playing a role. The actor while acting is completely identified with the role he is playing. He is no longer the person he was. Similarly, the mind may be identified with what it presents, and it behaves as if it is clear perception. But it is not based on true perception. The mind appears as if it is *cit*, or pure consciousness. This, however, is a misconception and not the truth. In the state of yoga, one has to be focused. There must be a connection on which that focus is based, so that the basis is real relationship. It is not the object that chooses the focus. I am the one who decides the focus.

H: So we have to establish a real and solid relationship, which allows us to focus. However, if I think about my experiences from psychotherapy and psychoanalysis, then I realize that we cannot assume this will happen right at the beginning. There are memories from the past, which may disturb this relationship and our capacity to focus. In psychoanalysis, we feel that there is a world inside us fueled by memories from our childhood, when we believed in the power of magic and dreams. Many people are so caught up in these dreams and desires that they are constantly disappointed. Advertising, for example, plays on this and suggests we can change ourselves simply by buying a certain product. Although we rationally know that this is not true, there is a "childish" and less conscious state within us that believes in these myths. This is what marketing slogans play on. Many people believe that they will become a new person if they find a new partner. When they experience the truth, that this is not the case, they are severely disappointed, and they separate. They thus need again and again to find a new partner to continue to live out this dream.

Even mentally healthy and stable people are subject to memories and pictures from their past. So we can assume that our ability to meditate or to concentrate on an object is curtailed. The mind is activated by its own structures and deceives itself. How can we deal with this?

D: The mind is like a wild horse. It has to be calmed, looked after, and tamed. It is not easy. That is why relationship in yoga is so important. Nowadays this is so difficult.

H: Sigmund Freud also used this image of a wild horse to describe our psychological structures. Freud saw a person's ego as the small rider on the wild horse of our instincts, which express the power and energy of the unconscious.

D: A good friend of mine from the West once beautifully described how psychoanalysis helped her: "I need a relationship. But I only see my yoga teacher once every six months. In psychoanalysis, I see my analyst twice a week. While I am lying on the couch, I am alone, but the analyst is sitting behind me. So I am not alone. I can feel free and I am in touch with him at the same time." I have seen how it helped this person; she changed so much. I saw her "standing up" after psychoanalysis. I can see how people after analysis are far more attentive and mature in yoga than before analysis. I think people in the West should do this to work on their mind.

The next sutra also speaks about the mind's activities:

> *vṛttayaḥ pañcatayyaḥ kliṣṭākliṣṭāḥ*
> There are five activities of the mind. Each of them can cause problems, and each can be beneficial. (YS I.5)

The mind has two sides: it can be very useful, and it can create great problems. It may help us to come out of something, or it may disturb and lock people up. A friend compared the mind to money. It can do much good for society, but people can also get addicted to money. Can you give another example?

H: Thought helps us to understand what moves us or causes us pain. Those who are suffering from feeling down can work with the help of a psychoanalyst to try to find the connections that are causing them to feel bad and that lead to feelings of sadness or depression. For example, let's look at the case of a patient of mine who came to an appointment suffering from severe depression and without the will to continue living. This person could not explain the severity of his depression. Later, this person briefly mentioned that he recently visited a doctor who told him that he might need a hip operation.

This patient was young and athletic and liked to be active. At the same time, he had a great deal of respect for authority and didn't dare ask for a specific diagnosis. He just imagined that in the future he would have to live with an artificial hip. He became so stuck in this way of thinking that it did not even occur to him to research the problem and ask his doctor for alternatives. He merely fantasized further, in part unconsciously, and this went so far that he became depressed and even lost the will to go on living. His thinking became self-fulfilling and showed him an outcome that was no longer connected to reality. When he began to discuss these fantasies with me, he came to see how his own thinking unconsciously established certain outcomes and prevented him from actually exploring what his real state was. Through conscious reflection, he became aware of the fact that there was the option to get more information. This example shows that thought can serve as a hindrance as well as an aid, depending on the level at which this thinking occurs.

At the beginning of his research, Freud viewed the human psyche as a machine that was able to regulate itself. Today, we might use computers for this analogy. They may help enormously if they work correctly, but not if they don't. If we are not able to master this tool, we may get into a real mess. The computer can provide valuable data or false data, depending on whether it works correctly and whether or not I am able to use it correctly.

D: That is a good example. The mind presents the data of what we perceive. So its activities may be beneficial or create problems. The mind in itself is neutral; it all depends on its state.

In this sutra, Patañjali reduces all the activities of the mind to five categories:

> *pramāṇa-viparyaya-vikalpa-nidrā-smṛtayaḥ*
>
> The five activities are comprehension, misapprehension, imagination, deep sleep, and memory. (YS I.6)

- Accurate representation and understanding is *pramāṇa*.
- Wrong representation and understanding is *viparyaya*.
- Imagination is *vikalpa*.
- Deep sleep is *nidrā*.
- Memory is *smṛti*.

These are the five activities of the mind.

We begin with the description of the right representation of the world, through the mind, which is the seventh sutra:

> *pratyakṣānumānāgamāḥ pramāṇāni*
> Comprehension is based on direct observation of the object, inference, and reference to reliable authorities. (YS I.7)

Patañjali first mentions direct perception (*pratyakṣa*), on which everything is grounded. Initially, there is direct perception: seeing what is in front of us. For that, we have to be connected to what is in front of us. We should try to understand. The second step is inference (*anumāna*). Let's assume we smell smoke. We infer that something is burning or that someone is cooking. This is the immediate inference, based on our direct perception. So the second step is inference or logical interpretation. This is then followed by reference (*āgama*) to books and the like, if necessary.

I will give you another example. Once I lost my passport at the Frankfurt airport. First I looked in all the places I had been. Then I wondered if it had fallen in the toilet or been stolen. This was an inference. Only then did I approach the information desk. See, it was based on experience first (the loss of the passport); the next step was the interpretation. How would you see this in your profession?

H: In our profession, we try to see the person before we get information from elsewhere. We don't conduct any tests. We rely on what we see and experience. Seeing does not mean looking with the eyes only. It also means trying to experience the whole situation. We virtually live with the person, feel what that person feels and think what he or she thinks. Only after that do we conceptualize or interpret the person's problem. Then we might make connections to other cases or to things we remember. After that, we would establish a connection to theoretical knowledge and to that which we have studied. Initially, we always rely on our direct perception and on the feelings this generates.

Similarly, when we present a case study, we first start with the situation and the quality of relationship we have with the person. Then there may be some reasoning. Only after this will there be a link to theory. You see there are similarities. As you told me, yoga is on the *vijñānamaya* level—the level of individual personality. So every situation and every individual is unique.

D: Yoga underscores the importance of *pratyakṣa* (correct direct perception). Observation through the senses first, experience next, then inference, and finally theory. This is characteristic of yoga, which is a living experience.

H: Every psychoanalyst would agree with this. It is essential to be in touch with reality. This is not about stories from the past, but rather about a living experience between the patient and the analyst. For this, we need to establish a stable relationship with the patient.

D: *Pramāṇa* means "correct understanding." How does this come about? I spoke about three steps: I must have an interaction, I must see, and based on what I see, I must pursue and investigate. When I find something missing, I can consult a reference. Right understanding is not based on assumption. First we must observe (see, listen); we use the mind only when we are still not sure; finally, we refer to an authority.

This is different from Hinduism, where everything is taught as the ancient texts say. The text says it, so you must accept it. God is this because the book says it. Because how can we see God?

H: How do I recognize the limits of my capacity to infer? How do I know if I have correctly understood something? There must be something that tells me the limits of my understanding or knowing. People have a tendency to categorize experiences according to things they already know so that they don't have to deal with anything truly new. I can convince myself that I know something in order to avoid the fear of the unknown.

D: *Anumāna* is a very interesting word: *māna* means "to measure"; *anu* means "to continue to pursue" this measurement. So you have to stay with the object and come closer and closer to it. You must find out for yourself. You have to discover what food is—for example, that food is the source of everything. You can find an investigation like this in the Upaniṣads. Suppose a person is in the middle of an ocean. In that situation, breath becomes more important. So the more we pursue, the more we find. It is a question of patience and perseverance.

H: In psychoanalysis, we would say it is very important to stay in touch with the object. This means to establish a relationship, to maintain it, and to deepen it.

D: That is why *atha yogānuśāsanam* is said first, which means "I want experience." What is yoga by experience? *Anuśāsanam* means "let me have the experience my teacher had."

H: In our work as psychoanalysts, it is expected that a therapist has at some point undergone psychoanalysis him- or herself. This way, the therapist can better feel and understand the position the patient is in, and the patient knows that he or she is not alone with what is experienced during therapy. This principle of shared experience seems to be an important one regarding the learning process within the context of relationship. When we work with our patients, the greatest challenge is to take every complaint and problem seriously and at the same time to ensure that we avoid conceptualizing, especially when we know what they are describing from our own experience.

D: It is important to let the students have their own experiences. Think of the famous book by M. Scott Peck, *The Road Less Traveled.* The analyst merely asked his patient how he was managing. He pursued the topic, and after a few weeks the patient asked him, "Are you talking about time management?" The analyst said, "Yes, that is why I am here. I am glad you found it." The client had to first discover the topic for himself; only then could he begin to really think about time management. We have to base things on experience and insight, not what the book says.

H: This means the yoga teacher should realize the importance of sometimes not speaking, of remaining silent, so that the students' experiences are not spoiled. The students should have the opportunity to find out by themselves and to be creative.

This is also an important principle in psychoanalysis. Other therapeutic schools in fact criticize this and claim that we leave our patients alone too much. However, we feel that only those insights that the patient makes for him- or herself are truly valuable. This is one of the main reasons for the occasional silence of the psychoanalyst. I myself have often seen that silence is as precious as gold. But remaining silent is not always easy! It is so tempting to want to say something.

D: The Upaniṣads would never say that someone is on the wrong path. Rather, it is said, To pursue your goal, go further. Then little by little, find out. The teacher could say, "I know the answer," but instead he or she says, "Find out yourself." This is a kind of meditation.

H: In order to understand this better, does it now make sense to look at the concepts of wrong perception and its structure?

D: The eighth sutra says:

viparyayo mithyā-jñānam atad-rūpa-pratiṣṭham
Misapprehension is that comprehension that is taken to be correct until more favorable conditions reveal the actual nature of the object. (YS I.8)

Until we know the truth, we are not sure if what we see is correct or incorrect. But we assume it is correct. We proceed according to this perception, and sometimes we pay a price. When I lost my passport in Frankfurt, I assumed it had fallen in the toilet because I thought it had been in my pocket. But it had actually fallen in the coffee shop when I had hung my jacket on a chair. So until I went to the information desk and the lady there told me, "This passport was found in the coffee shop," I was under the wrong impression. This is what the sutra says: "Until we see the actual truth, we continue to believe that a misperception is in fact right understanding." Why does this happen? It is because of certain assumptions and memories. Sāṅkhya explains this in the following way:

1. When an object is too close, we cannot see it.
2. When something is too far, we cannot see it.
3. When the mind is agitated, we cannot see clearly.
4. When the senses are disturbed, we cannot see clearly.
5. When something is there, but there is an obstacle, how can we see it?
6. When two things look too similar, we don't know which is what.
7. When something is very strong and something else is very weak, the former prevails and the latter is not seen. How can we see the stars when the sun is shining?

H: This sounds very modern. It reminds me of the laws of perception as they were developed in Germany by Wolfgang Metzger and others in Gestalt psychology. They were the first ones to show that perception is not objective but is dependent on context. What we are able to see depends on psychological laws that are determined situationally.

You have made clear that this is also the understanding of yoga. A yogi would always question his own perception and continually check his own understanding. This makes sense since we are never able to perceive reality in its totality.

Within psychoanalysis, we would say that someone who is absolutely convinced that he or she knows the truth, without questioning this in any way, has a serious problem with reality. Fanatical conviction about something may even indicate a psychotic disorder, especially if someone is too identified with what he or she believes to be the truth. That individual is confusing personal perception with the truth. As I understand you now, we should always be in a position to question our perceptions. This seems to be a cross-cultural truth that spans both Indian philosophy and Western psychoanalysis.

D: The other factor is change. For instance, that which I see now is not that which it will be tomorrow. Just because I saw something yesterday, so I might say today, "I know what this is." We don't easily accept change, which nonetheless happens all the time. When we open our eyes too late, we get into trouble. The second chapter of the Yogasūtra points this out and contains important material on how to minimize this. *Viparyaya* is very powerful.

H: This same phenomenon is familiar to psychoanalysts. We know that it's natural to try as much as is possible to block out the unfamiliar and see only that which we recognize. We assume this is because people are afraid of that which they do not yet know because they cannot control it. One of the biggest challenges in psychoanalysis, for the patient as well as for the therapist, is to continually remain open to the unknown. This means that they must learn to face the fear of the unknown. I can only truly understand something that I experience for myself. To do this, I need to free myself from prejudice and preconceived opinions. This creates fear. The unknown can be very stimulating, but first it creates fear. We are used to seeing the world as if we knew everything. That makes things easier. At the same time, we have to live continually with the fear of the unknown. Would you accept the premise that our tendency to be too quick to "see the truth" of a situation is ultimately based on fear?

D: Yes. The Yogasūtra says the origins of *viparyaya* are *avidyā*, *asmitā*, *rāga*, *dveṣa*, and *abhiniveśa* (the *kleśas*). If these are not present, there is no distortion of reality. In chapter 1, sutra 5, Patañjali says that right understanding or wrong understanding can be bad for us or good for us (*kliṣṭa akliṣṭa*). For example, wrong understanding can be an eye-opener; it can teach us something. Many discoveries in science follow errors. Distortion happens because of wrong association. What is the use of all this? The use is, because of this you can discover who is the boss and who is not the boss. Unless something unpleasant happens, we will not look at ourselves. This is what is so positive about Patañjali. Don't feel upset with problems in life. Because of these problems, you may be able to open your eyes. A wise person learns from mistakes.

H: In psychoanalysis, there are no true and no false answers. We attempt to discover unconscious meaning without making any judgments. For this, it is very important to be able to let thoughts and statements simply stand without making an interpretation about their veracity. Truth, insofar as we can discover it at all, is revealed only at the end of a long period of treatment. So here I agree with you. It is very important for the patient to have a psychoanalyst who can bear the tension of not knowing. In this manner, the patient can identify with the attitude of his or her analyst and thus develop the ability to better tolerate the state of not knowing. Only when both patient and analyst develop the ability to tolerate this state of not knowing can they discover something new.

All these thoughts are possible only if there is an activity called imagination. In our discipline, we say imagination is the basis or the root of the mind. It is considered to be the origin of psychic growth. By sustaining imagination, mental development can be fostered, as we experiment and then check our concepts and impressions against reality.

D: That is very interesting. The next sutra is about imagination:

> *śabda-jñānānupātī vastu-śūnyo vikalpaḥ*
> Imagination is the comprehension of an object based only on words and expressions, even though the object is absent. (YS I.9)

The sutra says that imagination is knowledge without the facts. That knowledge might be based on words, but there is no reality. Fiction, like Harry Potter, is to be understood in this way. Imagination can be speculation, too. For instance, you and I want to present Western psychology and yoga through some examples. This too is imagination—it is a plan for the future, not reality. So imagination can help prepare something. Sometimes it is an obstacle—for example, when we want something undesirable. It is a mental activity, which is always there. It may arise through dreams, feelings, or emotions. Very often people project their imagination onto others; this is not reality. But there is a productive side to imagination. If something is to happen, there must first be the idea or imagination, followed by a wish. Then other parts of the realization can follow. Without ideas, there can be no creation.

H: In psychoanalysis, we invite our patients to produce as many fantasies as possible. We invite them to share their daydreams. By speaking to them and analyzing these pictures and fantasies, we can glean their mental structures, which show us the way the patient thinks and interprets the world. Once we know a patient's fantasies, we can better understand his or her unconscious wishes. Daydreaming is very close to the productions of dreams. The structures developed in daydreaming are often also found in normal dreams in a hidden form. By analyzing and understanding this, we may be able to help patients understand their unconscious thinking. From there we can infer their feelings and wishes. By observing their fantasies, we can also understand their concept of relationship. By investigating their imagination, we are thus able to show them their own unconscious intentions.

Once patients have a better understanding of themselves and their environment, they can see themselves as master of their mental products and become aware of what they are doing in the world. In fact, they can see how they largely shape their own inner, and even outer, world. This is an "awakening" of the person in psychoanalysis. As opposed to the Yogasūtra, we in the psychoanalytic community see imagination as a powerful tool to understand the thoughts, the emotions, and even the whole personality of our patients. In fact, Sigmund Freud described imagination as the very source of mental functioning. So in applied psychoanalysis, imagination is a very powerful tool for human understanding. Often, people suffer from their unconscious fantasies, because these can lead to fear and anxiety. In psychoanalysis, we therefore invite our patients to reveal their imagination or fantasies in order to deal with these structures. Once we have understood a fear-provoking fantasy, it becomes less likely to create fear in the future. This process of producing fantasies and imagination is very healthy, because it helps patients organize their emotions and inner pictures and give them a character or a shape that patients can understand.

When people suffer from psychosomatic diseases, they have fewer unconscious fantasies. In lieu of these fantasies, they develop actual physical symptoms. By encouraging them to produce their fantasies again, we can reduce psychosomatic symptoms. You see, in this topic of imagination and fantasy, the yoga of Patañjali and psychoanalysis are distinct. Each culture has developed this idea differently. Perhaps this is because yoga came about in a very different time compared with the relatively young field of psychoanalysis?

D: We talked of *vikalpa*—imagination. You gave an example of how you in analysis ask the client to imagine something, which I find very interesting. Shall we go to the next sutra?

> *abhāva-pratyayālambanā tamovṛttir nidrā*
> Deep sleep is when the mind is overcome with heaviness and no other activities are present. (YS I.10)

Let's follow the order of presentation of the activities of the mind. The first three are *pramāṇa* (right understanding), *viparyaya* (distorted perception), and *vikalpa* (imagination). All these take place in the present. Then Patañjali goes to the next state, which is deep sleep. This is a movement of mind, which takes place neither in the present nor in the past because it is dreamless. Deep sleep is thus between the two time periods. (The next sutra will deal with the past—memory. Before that, let us look at deep sleep.)

The Sanskrit word for this is *nidrā*. *Nidrā* means something that makes a person heavy. It is a time when there is no comprehension or understanding. When there is heaviness in the system, I cannot hear what you say. I cannot see you, although you are there. Suddenly there is darkness. So it is an activity of the mind, which is the absence of all other activities. It is neither right nor wrong perception, neither memory nor imagination. This is dreamless deep sleep. Patañjali says that suddenly in the mind a quality of darkness appears—*tamas*. The darkness also has a quality of heaviness. The system cannot be alert. This happens unconsciously.

There are two types of sleep in yoga. Apart from deep sleep, the other form is an effort that stops everything—this is a state of yoga. It is not darkness. In this other state, I have the power to withdraw into myself. I don't want to see or listen. I am only within myself. That is called *yoga nidrā*.

The other *nidrā*, which I mentioned first (deep sleep), is not because I *want* to sleep; it simply takes over. Suddenly the darkness takes over. Why, we don't know. Perhaps because of the type of food we eat. Something changes in the body. So in yoga, we talk about two types of *nidrā*.

H: It seems to me that the *nidrā* of sleep has two aspects. It has the aspect of heaviness, and it also has the aspect of giving up or letting go. If I am to sleep, I must be able to let go and have the confidence that I will wake up again. There is therefore a beneficial side to *nidrā*. I think the definition is very precise because the word *nidrā* signifies that all activity of the mind ceases. For instance, there should not be any fear, because if there is fear, the person will dream in order to cope with it. If there is a great deal of fear, the person will wake up or won't sleep at all.

D: Imagine that you don't sleep for several days.

H: I would go crazy!

D: Sleep is very important, but not at the wrong time and not in the wrong situation. Sleeping at the wrong time is not good for me. That is why Patañjali says one of the biggest obstacles in life is fatigue. In the Upaniṣads, sleep is defined differently from the Yogasūtra. Here, pure consciousness goes back to its source, like a child who goes back to its source where it is comfortable and nourished. That explains why, after sleep, a person often feels refreshed. Sleep is rest for the mind.

The Yogasūtra says that although there is an absence of activity, not everything is in a state of sleep. *Cit* is not asleep! This is why, when we wake up, we are able to say we slept well or badly. There is an observer even during sleep. This, as already mentioned, is *draṣṭā*.

There is a story about this in the Upaniṣads. A teacher had a student who wanted to know what that is which is always alert. The teacher suggested they go for a walk, so they set off. They saw a person lying down. The teacher asked the student whether he knew the person. "Yes, I know this person," replied the student. "Who is he?" "He is a carpenter." "Okay, can you call him?" The student called to him, "Hello, get up!" However, he did not wake up. "Carpenter, get up!" Again, there was no response. Then, can you guess what the teacher did? He took a stick and hit the person. Immediately the person woke up and shouted: "Who is it?" What is implied here is: this is me, and this is *cit*. If I am awake, *cit* will get in contact with the senses and the world. In sleep, *cit* is withdrawn. So by hitting the person, what happens?

H: The person comes into contact with something painful.

D: Exactly. The energy radiates and the person is awakened. We call this *prāṇa*. When *prāṇa* is withdrawn, there is sleep. When *prāṇa* extends, there is wakefulness. For example, during a dream, *prāṇa* is linked to the mind. So we can see something. In deep sleep, *prāṇa* is not linked to the mind. We are not aware of anything. Suppose *prāṇa* is linked to feet: even in sleep the person will walk. There are people who sleepwalk!

H: So *prāṇa* may be linked to different objects, even inner objects, for example, when we dream?

D: Yes. When *prāṇa* is linked to the mind and senses, then the senses are active.

H: *Prāṇa* is the whole system of energy and energetic processes?

D: Yes.

H: In psychoanalysis, we have a similar system; we call it "libido." This refers to a kind of energy that connects us to certain things. If we feel attracted to a person, we say that we have libidinous feelings for this person. This means that a certain kind of psychic energy is affecting us.

D: Really? That is interesting. We say that if there is no *prāṇa* in the leg, for example, the person will also have no sensation in the leg.

H: It may happen in reality that people don't feel parts of their body, but they are not injured or ill. We then say that this part of the body does not have libidinous connections.

D: My first son's godfather once had an accident and lost sensation in his fingers. He could not move them; he had become handicapped. He asked his wife to read him some books. He then became quite philosophical. One day his wife read him a book about *prāṇa*. She read to him, "Where *prāṇa* flows, there are sensations. When there is no *prāṇa*, there is no sensation. If you don't have sensation in any part of the body, visualize that *prāṇa* is going there."

He then began to visualize *prāṇa* going to his fingers. He tried this because physiotherapy had not helped. After two months, he had sensation in his fingers. And then slowly he could move his fingers. Then he came to me and his fingers recovered completely. *Cit* has such great impact. I am not saying you can heal all diseases like this. But it is possible. We know of people who because of emotional problems develop some paralysis.

H: Can we return to the phenomenon of sleep for a moment? If we want to sleep, we must be able to momentarily relinquish all our desires and links to other people and objects. Children, for example, sometimes can't sleep because they are afraid of giving up their hold on things. For them, it is not self-evident that their world will still be there on waking. Of course, at some point they are overcome by exhaustion and they fall asleep. So if we want to sleep easily, we must be confident that something will sustain us. We should feel secure and know that the world is reliable and will still be there when we wake up again.

Another aspect is the environment in which we currently find ourselves. Here we also need some kind of reassurance. We need to prevent current or past problems from holding us awake. This means that we should have an internal and an external environment where we find it easy to let go for sleep.

D: It is difficult for some people to close the files on the past! There's a story about a lady who wrote a book. Nobody would publish it. Finally, she found someone who would. The book became very popular, and she was happy. She was asked to do promotions for the book in different cities. But then something terrible happened. Her son had a car accident and was seriously injured. On the one hand, she had been invited to support her new publication. There was money and fame in the offering. On the other hand, her son was injured. She didn't know what to do. She spoke to her husband. He said, "It is your choice. You can't be in both places." It was very difficult for her. She felt anger that such a thing would happen to her when she had finally been presented with a great opportunity. Why at this moment? She hesitated about making this decision for a month. Finally, the husband said to her, "If something happens to your son while you are absent, you will regret it forever. The promotion you can do later. Your son needs you now." So she made the decision to stay with her son.

H: This example shows how hard it can be for people to let go of something they had been hoping for that would provide them with a better future. This is often due to a lack of trust in the inner world of the mind. We see this with children when they don't want to go off to bed. They try everything to put this off. They become completely fixed on external objects. They don't want to give anything up because they fear losing it. Marcel Proust describes this at the beginning of *Remembrance of Things Past*. He exactly describes his torturous memories of being brought to bed and fighting the process of falling asleep because he feared he would never see his mother again.

D: Let us look at the next sutra:

> *anubhūta-viṣayāsampramoṣaḥ smṛtiḥ*
> Memory is the mental retention of a conscious experience.
> (YS I.11)

The English word for *smṛti* is "memory." Patañjali says we remember that which had an impact on us. There is an incident that happened eighteen years ago that I still remember. I was traveling from India to Boston. As I had flown Swissair, I had only Swiss money. I was hungry. I went to the café in the airport's domestic terminal and asked for tea. When I gave Swiss money to the waitress, she said they did not take it. I told her I had no dollars and so I gave her back the tea. She asked me, "Where are you coming from?" I said, "I just arrived from India." "Oh," she said. "Was it a long flight?" "Yes, from Madras to Bombay, from Bombay to Zurich, and then Boston." You know what she said? "Have this tea, be my guest. Don't worry about the dollars." She insisted. Then she came back and said, "You can't just have tea. You should have some snacks, too." So she brought me some cake. "Be my guest. Don't worry. Just relax."

Two years later when I went to Boston again, I wanted to give her a gift from India. I went to the same café, but the manager said she had already left. This is memory. This experience had such an impact on me that I cannot forget it.

So this is how memory is presented. In life there is something happening at every moment except when we are in deep sleep. Certain things happen that we are linked to and are conscious of; this is never mechanical. This is why Patañjali says that experience has an impact and can never be lost.

There are two types of memory. One is an experience—like a sheet of paper; the second is creative. Some memories become the basis for creativity. Patañjali says that in dreams, memory is creative. While we are awake, memory takes in only what is happening. This is then based on experience.

H: How can memory create?

D: Take memory in the dream state and memory in the waking state. Memory in the former is a creative memory. When I see you, Hellfried, some things pass through my memory. Your first question to me was about change, for example. Once your car broke down when we met, you remember? These are facts. But in dreams something else happens. This is called *bhāva* memory. Memory is the seed, and it is from the seed that plants arise. That is why in dreams many things happen; this is because when we are in a dream state we have time for creativity. There is no hurry. While awake, on the other hand, we go constantly from one thing to the next.

H: Can you say that in dreams there is a mixture, or a union, between memory and imagination? Imagination might take over some part of memory and produce something new?

D: Yes. Agreed.

H: The examples you gave about memory, and the impact it has on our life and our consciousness, were about deep or moving experiences. You were in contact with someone who was able to give you something you needed. You were lost and then someone came and gave you something. So can we say that the impact of memory is related to emotional relationships, perhaps even with the first and most important relationship?

D: Yes, and this is not necessarily linked to time. Many things that happen again and again, we don't remember. Certain things happen for a moment, but they are never forgotten. From my time at university—I studied engineering for five years—I remember some incidents. I don't remember what I learned, but I remember incidents that appeared unimportant at the time.

H: Those things that touch us emotionally seem as if they happened yesterday.

D: Yes.

H: In psychoanalysis, we also say that unconscious memories are timeless. There is no notion of time in the unconscious. Does the Yogasūtra speak of the influence of memory on how we perceive the world, and then on how we act?

D: Yes. That is an important question. In India, we do everything with the right hand. Eating, welcoming. We are trained to do this. It is called "conditioning." When we do something again and again, it becomes like a reflex. Conditioning has a very strong relationship to memory. We call conditioning *saṁskāra*. You recall that the Sanskrit word for memory is *smṛti*. *Saṁskāra* and memory are strongly linked. Although in India we eat with our hands, when I go abroad, I use a knife and fork. Automatically, memory is provoked and my system shifts, because I have had that training or experience. Different situations trigger different *saṁskāras*, and this conditioning helps us recall memory. Here in India, for example, I hardly remember German. But after I spend two days in Germany, suddenly terms like *Guten Morgen* and *Auf Wiedersehen* come to me.

Memory is provoked both by conditioning and by the environment. Sometimes it happens after months or years. There is a beautiful sutra in the fourth chapter: "Memory and latent impressions are strongly linked. This link remains even if there is an interval of time, place, or context between similar actions." (YS IV.9)

H: You describe three aspects of memory. One is linked to emotions, another is based on *saṁskāra* (conditioning), and then there are memories linked to specific situations. Different situations provoke different memories. Similarly, in psychoanalysis we have found different kinds of memory.

In fact, we have also identified a fourth kind of memory in psychoanalysis, which we can call "the past in the present." We mean by this that the activation of unconscious memories may become current in a specific situation. A person may suddenly act as he or she did twenty or thirty years ago. For instance, let's take a grown man who has completed his studies and is about to start work as a teacher. He gets along well with his pupils, and his ability to teach is exemplary. However, he cannot work as a teacher because he cannot bear being with his colleagues in the staff room. Older teachers cause him so much fear that he can only flee. They cause him to regress to the state of being a terrified young boy who can do nothing but run away.

We call this kind of inappropriate reaction to a situation "acting out." This behavior strongly resembles patterns of behavior established in the past with parents, teachers, and so on. It is a kind of repetition; the past becomes present. But people suffering from this do not recognize it as such. So our work is to make them aware that they are reacting and behaving on the basis of memory and not according to actual reality. We also call this kind of behavior "scenic memory" because it repeats whole situations as if an old movie is playing again and again. Does this model exist in yoga philosophy as well?

D: Yes. *Saṁskāra* (conditioning) is a very strong factor in our life. Though I can intellectually assess the situation, what determines my behavior and communication is strong *saṁskāras*, deep patterns within me. *Saṁskāra* is the seed, and memory is the flower. If you want to reduce negative *saṁskāra*, you need to create new patterns. As the latter becomes stronger, the former becomes weaker. We cannot destroy *saṁskāra*, or memory. But we can introduce new ones. The old memory or pattern is not dead, it is just less effective.

The fruits of our actions are also responsible for the revival of memory and *saṁskāra*. We do something and we get something. The result of action affects our memory, too. Let me cite an example. Suppose I invest money in stocks; if the stocks go down in value, I lose money, get depressed, and can't forget it. Another example relates to our environment: Let us imagine I am going on an eight-hour plane journey somewhere. I reach a different place, the situation changes. The state of mind changes, too. Because of the *guṇas*, *rajas*, *tamas*, and *sattva*, the mind is not always the same. Unexpectedly, certain memories and conditioning can suddenly surface. So now we see there are four factors in the revival of conditioning and memory: various causes, results of actions, environment, and the state of mind. If the mind changes, something changes. Suddenly people change, they get depressed even though everything is fine. Why is this? Because of some change in the mind. (YS IV.11)

The way we function, the way we think, is based mostly on conditioning. This is why in the Upaniṣads *saṁskāra* is in the *vijñānamaya* level. It is called *mahat*. This is not due only to the way we are brought up. It could be genetic, but it is individual. In India, we say it is not genetic. We say it is because of experiences when we were young. Not necessarily in this life, but in past lives. In Hinduism, there exists the concept of previous lives and of the soul taking birth many times. In the Yogasūtra, there is no such reference. The Yogasūtra merely says that something that happened previously will have consequences in the future (YS II.12).

H: In psychoanalysis, when we work with patients our premise is that they are caught in concepts of the past. They are imprisoned by unconscious memories. We try to understand this along with them. We try to make the patient understand how some behavior stems from the past. And by understanding how a person in the present behaves as if it were the past, he or she can be freed from this repetition. When that person becomes able to see and feel things as they truly occur in the present, it is a liberation. But as you already mentioned, an intellectual explanation is not enough. The person must experience all the unconscious feelings and emotions from this past occurrence and understand them. For this, the analyst needs a strong relationship with the patient, with a deep level of trust between them.

D: This is very interesting. Let me give you an example. A woman suffered from a lot of anxiety. This was common in her family. Fear was a strong theme: fear of death, financial insecurity, going out alone at night. Tremendous fear. She got married to someone from a family that was different. When he said, "Let us go to the cinema," she said, "I can't go to the cinema. It is so dark in the theater." So he took her to a movie during the day. After a month he took her to an evening show and then to the night show. After a year she was not scared of going to the cinema at any time of day. But she still had other fears. She was afraid of traveling on a moped at night. She was frightened of dead bodies. (In India, dead bodies are exhibited in the open.) Her husband told her, "Sit behind me on the moped. If you see a dead body, just close your eyes." So she got accustomed to closing her eyes whenever she saw a funeral procession.

But this did not solve the problem of what would happen if someone in the family died. She would not go to see the body. After a while, she decided she could go to see the body, but when her grandmother died, she began having nightmares. She also feared flying in airplanes, so her husband had to travel alone.

Now, fifteen years later, she is no longer troubled by the sight of a dead body. She is even able to fly alone. This is an example of transformation by relationship. The anxiety may be still there, but it gets no nourishment, and the opposite reaction is nourished instead through her strong relationship with her husband.

H: May we assume she was exposed to very stressful situations when young? Her fear could be explained by this. Overcoming her fears with the help of her husband was a late development in her life. It was not easy, but it was possible. Without this relationship, she would not have changed.

D: I have seen her sisters. They are still scared. None of them have a comparable relationship.

H: Could we say the most important factors to effect change on memory are emotion and relationship, in both yoga and psychoanalysis?

D: Yes. There must be love. You cannot order someone to change, but you should believe it can happen. It should be done with love and positive emotions. It takes time. This, I feel, is the biggest defect in yoga today. Though yoga deals with relationship, it often is not through a significant relationship. Relationship is not just preaching.

Yesterday I received a fax from a woman I know. I was touched by the way it was presented, with flowers and pictures! There should be feelings. That is missing in many forms of yoga today. I am sorry to say it, but without real relationship, no transformation is possible.

2

What Steps Must We Take to Change?

YOGASŪTRA, CHAPTER TWO (*sādhana-pādaḥ*)

T.K.V. Desikachar: The first sutra of the second chapter reads as follows:

> *tapaḥ-svādhyāyeśvara-praṇidhānāni kriyā-yogaḥ*
> The practice of yoga must reduce both physical and mental impurities. It must develop our capacity for self-examination and help us to understand that in the final analysis, we are not the masters of everything we do. (YS II.1)

This chapter deals with the importance of yoga and how it can be achieved. It is the why and the how. In the discussions on the first chapter, I defined yoga as being completely in the present moment, sustaining a relationship. In such a state, something special can be discovered.

That which we must do to achieve this goal is called *sādhana*; the effort needed to reach it is called *kriyā-yoga*. *Kriyā* means "to act" and also "action." Action is required to experience the state of total attention. *Kriyā* has three elements: *tapas*, *svādhyāya*, and *Īśvara-praṇidhāna*.

Tapas is the identification of impurities in our psychosomatic system that cause problems. It is similar to an awakening: the discovery and use of a potential that is not being tapped. Take the example of a simple cooking pot. It might in fact be a good pot, but because it is dirty or rusty, it cannot be used immediately. First, the dirt has to be removed. Note that there are two processes here—noticing of the dirt and its removal. We have to find a way to remove the dirt. Once that is done, the pot is ready for use. *Tapas* is the identification of impurities in our system that cause many of our problems, and then, step by step, the removal of those impurities. These may be of a physical, emotional, or intellectual nature. We do not live through life maintaining the innocence of a baby. Over time, things happen that may affect or change our life as we are exposed to many influences. The cooking pot does not remain new. Similarly, our system is not new or clean. And cleaning it requires discipline. This is the meaning of *tapas*.

Svādhyāya means that we should verify constantly where we are, look at ourselves, question ourselves. We need to "check the pot" and, to continue with the metaphor, ensure, for example, that certain chemicals used won't destroy it. We need to ask, "Am I the same person I was ten years ago? Has this effort brought any change in me?" We must continually question and investigate ourselves. This attitude of self-examination is called *svādhyāya*.

Īśvara-praṇidhāna is tremendously important because it describes the inner attitude in which yoga should take place. When we attempt something, we cannot predict whether or not it will succeed in the way we want. Anything may happen. Life is difficult and often a mystery. We should not get upset or lose our temper when the results we seek are not attained. So this attitude of putting in the effort, accepting certain types of failures, and continuing to pursue a goal is called *Īśvara-praṇidhāna*. For someone who has faith in God, *Īśvara-praṇidhāna* could mean asking a higher force: "God, I have put in my effort. I now ask you to share your grace so that it will help me succeed. I myself cannot judge the result of my actions."

In pursuing a goal, one should first identify what is getting in the way of attaining it; one should try slowly and carefully to remove these obstacles, constantly questioning one's own role and being open to either success or failure. The outcome is not in our hands. Sometimes good things happen, sometimes the unexpected. We put in effort with hope. *Īśvara-praṇidhāna* means to accept this and not to be disappointed when there is failure. Continue to pursue your goals, but acknowledge that you are not a perfect being. This is the spirit of yoga and of yoga practice leading to its highest goal: complete attention.

Hellfried Krusche: I feel there is great wisdom in this sutra that doesn't even require further comment. In psychoanalysis, we don't ask people to do *tapas* in the sense of cleansing or purifying. We don't have this concept of "impurities" in the psychophysical system. Instead, we assume there are internal, unconscious conflicts we would like to bring to conscious awareness. We attempt to meet the patients in their current state of mind. We motivate them by establishing a relationship, we think they will identify with our way of working, and we hope they can develop continuity with us for some time. We don't ask patients to do anything specific apart from coming to appointments regularly and paying the fees for the sessions. Even this can be difficult and perhaps resembles *tapas* in your system: asking people to make an effort.

When it comes to *svādhyāya*, however, this is the most important part of our work. We try to help people understand what they are doing and why they are doing it at the very moment they are engaging in a particular behavioral pattern. When they are with us, we try to mirror how they behave with themselves and with us on an emotional level. For this, it is essential to have confidence, trust, and a good relationship. Together we try to understand where they are now in their relationship with us and in what direction they want to develop.

Regarding the last concept, *Īśvara-praṇidhāna*, I want to stress that this point of view is at the center of new approaches to psychoanalysis. We describe it differently, however. Psychoanalysts believe that there is a strong tendency in mentally disturbed people to perceive the world as they would like it to be. The main goal in working with these patients is to achieve a relationship in which they can tolerate the realization that the analyst is different from them, that we see things differently and that we live differently. Patients are thus encouraged to develop tolerance. A capacity to relinquish control over oneself and over others is one of the most important results of successful psychoanalytic therapy. In this I see a strong similarity to the concept of *Īśvara-praṇidhāna*: to accept that certain things can't be changed, that the analyst leads his or her own life, that you can't change your boss or your wife, that reality is different from what you expected it to be. This fundamental realization signifies successful transformation through psychoanalysis.

Let's take the example of a woman who begins psychoanalysis only because she privately hopes to later marry her analyst. With this secret goal in mind, she is willing to do whatever is needed, even become healthy again. It's a great shock for her when she discovers that her analyst is already married. She then wants to end her treatment. The main goal in continuing her treatment is to make it clear to her that her analyst lives and feels differently from what she had previously assumed. Only when she realizes this will she be able to find a suitable partner for herself. Being able to continue to work with her analyst and accepting that her relationship to him has boundaries that she can't alter are intertwined.

This is the beginning of a truly deep inner change for this patient. So we see here some similarities between psychoanalysis and yoga.

D: When you ask a client to come to appointments on time, and make a commitment to see you regularly as a psychoanalyst, and agree to pay the fees, and accept that the relationship with you remains within the psychoanalysis and does not extend beyond that, then I agree: this is a form of *tapas*.

H: In our work, besides *tapas*, there is also something similar to what you have called *Īśvara-praṇidhāna*. It is not explicitly named or conceptualized as such. But in a certain sense, when analyst and client meet, there is a kind of selection. A patient seeks out an analyst with whom that patient believes he or she can work well. In a similar manner, when an analyst proposes that a particular patient undergo analysis with him or her, it is important that the analyst believes in the capacities of the patient to overcome difficult experiences. The analyst must assume that this patient has the ability to give certain things up or to endure some frustration. This can even be something trivial, such as the fact that in big cities, for instance, it takes time to get through traffic to meet with the analyst.

For years, I met with a patient starting at 7:00 a.m. He simply was not able to come at any other time. This required sacrifice and commitment on both sides. But in the end it worked out well, and the patient made excellent progress.

You see, we work with people who need help because they don't know how to continue with their lives. In yoga, you see people who want to further develop their lives. In general, people who practice yoga are not involved in a current conflict. In general, they are more stable than patients. The goal of yoga extends beyond the goals of psychoanalysis. In psychotherapy, we aim to overcome internal conflicts and develop the ability to engage in long-term, satisfying relationships with other people. The goal of yoga is geared more toward taking an already well-functioning mental condition and moving it toward an even higher goal.

D: There is, however, a current problem with yoga. Many people don't know how they should really practice. It appears to me there is a problem with the way yoga is taught; something seems missing. As it is presented nowadays, it is not very clear how one can practice yoga. There are so many different schools, and every school appears to emphasize different things. Is it yoga if you follow certain training courses, read books, and attend seminars on different topics? Is this yoga as described here in the second chapter: *tapaḥ-svādhyāyeśvara-praṇidhānāni*?

Today, yoga students read lots of notes, do some postures, meditate on various topics. However, it is not very clear whether this is happening at a level higher than what you have been describing in psychoanalysis. In our tradition, the strength of yoga derives its power from the relationship between the teacher and the student. If the relationship is not there, then yoga has no meaning.

I recently called a student of mine because I wanted to see him. Although he is a busy and important person, he said, "Your wish is my command." This is the way he sees the teacher. So he said, "I will cancel something and be there at 7:30 p.m." I was so touched. I have never taken advantage of my influence, but this illustrates something. For me, the connection between the student and the teacher is the foundation. Techniques are superficial structures, something that is put on the surface. But I am not sure whether such fundamental relationships still exist in the contemporary world of yoga.

H: Perhaps this could be described as the special quality of a good relationship.

D: The confidence this student had in me came as a result of the success of the work we did together. For this work, one has to have competence. It is not enough merely to do some postures. We should know our students, and we should understand their mental or psychological structures. We must then design a practice just for them and observe them doing it. As soon as they start to practice in this way regularly, there will be results. These are some of the factors leading to a deep relationship.

There is an example of a yoga teacher who recently said to me, "I don't know why I do yoga. I could also do different things." So I had a chat with her. She always appeared tense. I asked, "Why are you so nervous?" Then I said, "If you are so nervous, do you think you can be a very effective teacher? Shouldn't you do something to reduce this nervousness?" She replied, "When I get enough sleep, I am okay." I asked, "Are you sure that you sleep well when you are constantly so agitated?" Then she told me that one of her previous yoga school partners left her school and opened a new school right next door. This created tension. "Don't you think it is even more important for you to be quiet and relaxed, because next door your former partner is competing with you?" She agreed. "I need to do something for myself. Can you teach me?" She wanted to learn. After a few weeks, she said she understood. I then found someone to continue to teach her. She is now continuing with this teacher and is very committed.

H: Sometimes after having worked intensely for a longer period of time with a patient, the quality of the relationship changes in such a way that these patients appear very familiar to us. We have some patients who see us during their psychoanalytic treatment three or more times per week, and this can continue over several years. Imagine how intense this relationship becomes! If I then meet a former patient years after the end of treatment, I feel joyful. It feels like resuming a loving relationship. This is something very special. When I am awaiting them, I feel my heart beating a little faster. This is mostly the case in longer-lasting therapies with several sessions every week and where significant changes took place. This deep emotional connection, which can be present even years after termination of therapy, seems to me to be the energy of transformation. I can imagine that this quality of relationship is also a central factor in yoga, and I share your opinion.

I would like to illustrate this with an example. Recently I led a seminar for yoga teachers. There was a woman, a very successful yoga teacher, who wanted to see me in a one-to-one meeting. She told me that although she had a yoga school, she had not been able to do her own practice for more than two years. She was facing personal problems that she couldn't overcome. When she tried to practice yoga, all her sadness would come up and she was afraid it would overwhelm her. She was a very bright and beautiful woman, but she had a rigid appearance, and behind this she was very depressed. All her strength and energy went into maintaining her beautiful facade. She was so afraid of her depression that she no longer dared do yoga because this put her in contact with those feelings. She also had had a medical examination and the blood tests showed that her immune system seemed about to collapse. She was afraid of falling seriously ill.

She felt trapped and asked for help. We arranged for her to do therapy with me on condition that she resumed her regular yoga practice. She agreed to this, although she was still quite fearful. After a few weeks of treatment, her appearance changed. Her depression surfaced, she no longer looked so "walled in"; instead, she now looked like someone who had a shadow. She spoke to me about her suicide attempts many years back. By building up a relationship, she had the courage to face her depression and resume yoga. She was able to allow herself to cry during our appointments. After such sessions, she told me how good it felt to let go. Some weeks later, her blood tests improved dramatically. Then we worked for some time to tackle her depression.

During the third year of her treatment, she met a partner and they moved into a new home together. She now appears more open and less "shiny"; she is a beautiful person who is able to stand on her own two feet, with stable and loving connections in the environment in which she lives.

It is obvious that the yoga practice she had been doing was no longer enough to help her solve her problems. There was no yoga teacher available where she lived who was able to understand her sufficiently. At the same time, resuming her practice was an enormous factor in speeding and aiding her recovery.

Again and again I have observed that psychotherapy patients who practice yoga at the same time are able to develop more quickly and at a deeper, more fundamental level. We need yoga teachers who are able to help people when they are in emotional crises. This involves, I believe, the ability to understand people at this level of relationship.

To come back to our topic: Therapy itself was a kind of *tapas* for this woman. It involved courage and determination to open up and also to resume her yoga practice. The emergence of her fears and emotions, and speaking about her current state, was *svādhyāya*. She had been in a difficult situation, and at the outset she could not have known that the result would be to help her come out of her depression. She trusted in the process of this work. This is a variation of *Īśvara-praṇidhāna*.

D: This sutra talks about three things: first we have to apply some effort; then we must review, reflect, and question ourselves; and finally there should be openness regarding expectations and results.

In yoga, attention, relationship, and the ability to be present to what is happening (*samādhi bhāva*) are all crucial. Sometimes I have people in front of me who are not really present because they are preoccupied with something else. By understanding this, we can perhaps discover that which is within us, that which is between us, and that which prevents us from seeing clearly.

How does this happen? Something like a cloud can cover up our clarity or cause it to vanish. These clouds are called *kleśas*. *Kleśa* refers to something that causes suffering and by doing so prevents clear perception.

The second sutra in the second chapter points out that not all suffering is due to external factors:

> *samādhi-bhāvanārthaḥ kleśa-tanū-karaṇārthaś ca*
> Then such practices will be certain to remove obstacles to clear perception. (YS II.2)

It can be caused by something within us. For example, yesterday I went out for a meal. Someone was sitting next to me. He was upset because it was raining ten miles south of his home, and he was complaining that it was not raining on his property. Instead of being happy about the much needed rain and thinking about the joy of the plants where it was raining, he was unhappy. In his case, suffering was caused by excessive selfishness or self-centeredness. The sutras emphasize that it is important for us to reduce these internal factors that block us.

The next sutra expands on these *kleśas*:

avidyāsmitā-rāga-dveṣābhiniveśāḥ kleśāḥ
The obstacles are misapprehensions, confused values, excessive attachments, unreasonable dislikes, and insecurity. (YS II.3)

- *avidyā*—misapprehension, wrong understanding
- *asmitā*—egotism, self-centeredness, false identity
- *rāga*—temptation, addiction, excessive attachment
- *dveṣa*—hatred, rejection, unreasonable dislike
- *abhiniveśa*—fear, especially fear of death, insecurity

These are the obstacles that obstruct correct perception.

H: So if I understand you correctly, the *kleśas* are obstacles that are always present and can always affect people. So I have to simply accept that they exist.

D: A cousin of mine had stomach pains. However, he refused to see a doctor. Only when complications arose did he relent. The doctor asked, "Why didn't you come earlier? Now it is too late." One month later, my cousin died of cancer. Sometimes we can't accept that we need to seek help. When someone comes to you for help, at least he or she has recognized a need. Some people are ashamed to accept help or to share their problems. The consequences can be grave.

H: Fear of illness seemed to play an important role in your cousin's case. This fear caused him not to take his symptoms seriously. Perhaps he was also afraid of accepting help from others, thus losing his independence. Giving up his independence became more important to him than his own life. We call behavior like this "denial." He was no longer able to differentiate the essential from the nonessential.

D: That is why the sutra says that the first step toward wisdom is recognizing that one is in trouble and having clarity about this. The second step is acknowledging that the trouble has a cause. The third step is accepting that one must come out of the troubled situation, and for this to happen, effort needs to be applied. The fourth step is deciding to put in this effort, whatever happens. This is great practical wisdom.

Let me repeat:

1. "I am in trouble, no doubt about it."
2. "I am in trouble because of what happened to me."
3. "I must put in some effort so that I will be free from that."
4. "What exactly shall I do? Yes, I am ready to do that."

Why do we suffer? We suffer because something in us causes us to suffer. How it came to this, we cannot say, but our suffering has a source. Patañjali calls it *avidyā. Avidyā* comes from the Sanskrit word *a* plus *vidyā. Vidyā* comes from the Sanskrit word *vid*, which means "to know." There are many words that are derived from *vid*, like *veda*—knowledge. *Avidyā* means the opposite of this. It refers to a kind of "knowing" that is fundamentally different from what actually is. In other words, the information driving our actions may be misinformation.

Here is a nice example. This microphone you use has a stand. Up until today we had not noticed the stand. That is *avidyā*. Today, for the first time, we noticed it. That is *vidyā*. *Avidyā* can be caused by not knowing something at all, or believing something to be different from what it really is. This happens because all of our perceptions come through the mind, and they are thus mixed with the patterns or "colors" of the mind. The "color" therefore stems from the mind and not the object. It is as if we are wearing sunglasses and then we see some clouds. Naturally, they appear dark. But this is not the clouds, it is the sunglasses. We forget that and think it is really dark. We assume that what we see is reality and proceed based on that. If we knew the color of the mind, we could subtract that and then we would know what the object was really like.

H: When we do psychoanalysis, we try to understand the patient's mind by working through emotional experiences with the patient. Through this process, old patterns of experiencing emotions and feelings are revealed. By doing this repeatedly, the patient may become aware of tendencies to see and do things in certain ways. We thus sensitize patients to the fact that there is always some influencing factor that is unknown and of which they were probably unaware. This new awareness of things that were previously unconscious is one of the most important results of psychoanalysis. From this we gain the capacity to question our own behavior, to ask ourselves, "What I am doing here, and what exactly is it I am perceiving?"

D: How do you help your patients to discover their earlier lives—that is, uncover experiences from childhood?

H: This is a key question. As you have already mentioned, it is very important to establish an emotional relationship with the patient. People hide emotional experiences from childhood in their everyday emotions. We try to activate this emotional memory within the context of our relationship. The past is then expressed in an encoded way, with allusions, within the therapeutic setting. Our task is to perceive these encoded messages, to meet them with our own feelings, and then to use our professional knowledge to decode them. This is what we call "emotional understanding." We can then make very specific hypotheses about the patient's early childhood, which we can verify and further clarify in discussions with the patient.

As soon as I feel I have understood the issue, I share my insights with the patient. Then I ask if he or she has experienced similar feelings in other situations, and then we use this new perspective to look at the patient's current problems. After several years of therapy, it is often possible to formulate the main problem of a patient so precisely that it can be stated in two lines. From this, one can deduce and understand a person's problems and likely behavior.

For example, let's take a patient who grew up without a father. His mother was very depressed because she was alone, without any help whatsoever. The patient had extraordinary skills. He was highly intelligent, but he also had very severe symptoms. He couldn't perceive the world correctly. He sometimes felt he saw the world around him in only two dimensions. For five years during therapy, he demonstrated to me that he was able to survive in a number of different situations. He showed this in very different fields such as in sports, in financial matters, even in his job. At the same time, it became clear to me that he wanted to find out whether or not I would remain calm and continue to give him a sense of security. In this way, he brought an element of his problem into our relationship.

I then formulated the hypothesis that he might have been traumatized by the fact that his mother wasn't able to provide him with a safe and secure environment in which he could grow up without fear or tension. It turned out that his mother suffered from serious mental illness, and she was unable to deal with his vitality. In fact, she was afraid of him. I came to the conclusion that he was forced to be extremely attentive from the first moments of his life because he feared he could fall into an empty chasm and that his mother would not be able to help him. He was forced to adopt this behavior as a small child in order to survive. Over time, this hypothesis became more and more consistent. To the extent that the patient began to understand himself better, he became able to accept that I might be interested in him and his development. He began to trust me more and more. Some symptoms disappeared. For more than forty years he had lived in a situation of stress without being aware of it. Improvement came with awareness. Without knowing it, he had also developed the tendency to withdraw from people and to observe them from a distance. He did this especially when he was afraid of something. With his fear, he also became afraid of losing contact with the world to the point of falling out of it. The more he became aware of his stress and his tendencies to avoid contact and emotions, the more he was able to recognize and understand himself. Finally, he was able to overcome some of his severe symptoms, which were actually a part of his withdrawal. We found the structure of his mental functioning, and by doing so, his condition improved. He later got married and became a father.

D: This was a very impressive example! In India, we now have a problem that we call "guru business." People tend to be too dependent on their "gurus." A former president of India was so attached to his guru that he cried for days when his guru died. He cried like a child, and he was the president of a country with more than one billion people. There is an element of slavery in this, and it is not good. When my teacher died, I didn't cry. I told people who asked that when my teacher was alive, I used to see him for an hour or two every day, and now my teacher is in me, he is with me. For many people this is not clear. The difference is that you can feel *for* a person, but you should not feel *with* a person. The latter destroys people. There must be a certain distance; you must be able to stand on your own two feet.

H: In such cases, could the relationship itself become what you call *avidyā*?

D: Dependent people will do anything they are asked to do. They stop thinking and go from ignorance to deep darkness. They want to ask their guru for help on any decision.

H: It seems like childish behavior, a resistance to growth and adulthood, to insist on maintaining this childishness.

D: This, however, is not what yoga intends. Yoga expects us to stand on our own two feet. That is why yoga would say that if I want to learn swimming, I need a teacher, but the aim is ultimately to swim by myself. Then I should also become able to teach others.

H: If *avidyā* is to be reduced, we have to stand up and have our own experiences. I think *avidyā* is present whenever there are strong emotions. So how can I know when there is *avidyā* and when not?

D: In the past, something happened and I suffered. Now the same thing happens and I don't suffer. There is a beautiful story of a very old Zen master sitting under a tree and meditating. He sees a hungry tiger, so weak it is not even able to walk. He approaches the tiger, thinking, "I will offer myself to the tiger." He goes even closer, but the tiger is too weak to eat him. So he begins to cut his fingers, his arm, his feet, and give them to the tiger, who slowly eats the flesh. The tiger gains strength and then eats the man entirely.

This story is a metaphor about nonattachment. I feel this man has overcome one of the deepest attachments. He was old. By doing what he did, he was able to serve the tiger! He had no fear about offering himself. One of the problems of *avidyā* is attachment to this and that.

The story continues. After a while, the master's students come to see him and can't find him. Then they see some clothes and they know a tiger has eaten the master. They decide to kill the tiger and prepare to do this. Then they find a small sheet of paper on which is written, "Don't kill the tiger. It is a tigress and it is pregnant. I want to save her babies." They look around and see the tigress with her cubs. Tears come into their eyes!

To think that you have no *avidyā* is the biggest *avidyā*!

After speaking about *avidyā*, let us now turn to the other *kleśas*. Just as *avidyā* is false apprehension, *asmitā* is false identification. *Rāga* is temptation in the expectation of pleasure, which can include addiction. *Dveṣa* is hatred due to negative experiences such as pain and rejection in the past that troubles the memory. Finally, *abhiniveśa* is fear, mainly fear of death. This last element is somewhat of a mystery. Even though we know intellectually that we are not going to live forever and that everything is not in our hands, we still fear death. Even wise people suffer from this. According to yoga, this fear stems from some idea of death that we have, either intellectually or emotionally. We are insecure because we want to survive. We are attached to life because we don't know what will happen when we die. Patañjali says this is the cause of our mental distortion, our lack of clarity and suffering.

H: It seems to me that *abhiniveśa* is pervasive on several evolutionary levels. Fear of death appears to be active in every living being, from simple animals to human beings. We also find examples of *dveṣa* and *rāga* in mammals. These animals show tendencies to react to certain situations and associated behavioral patterns. Behavioral science carries out experiments in this field and studies the behavior of animals; it sets up contrived situations to test likes and dislikes. Behavioral therapy has successfully applied many of these insights and developed therapeutic approaches for human beings based on these insights.

In general, I think it is important to see that yoga recognizes so many elementary motivation systems. I would call them fear, greed, and rejection. They are fundamental motivations, but the way they may be organized seems to be determined by our sense of "I" (*asmitā*), the way a person conceptualizes and understands him- or herself. So I think we have to focus on *asmitā*. We know that there are compulsions, that there is fear. How the human being is able to cope with these is important. But *asmitā* seems the most typically human trait. Only human beings are able to self-identify. Animals cannot do this. Shall we therefore focus on *asmitā*?

D: The sixth sutra in the second chapter discusses *asmitā*. I suggest we discuss this first and then come back to the two previous sutras, 4 and 5.

The sixth sutra says:

> *dṛg-darśana-śaktyoḥ ekātmatevāsmitā*
> False identity results when we regard mental activity as the very source of perception. (YS II.6)

There are certain qualities in consciousness. *Dṛg-darśana-śaktyoḥ* means "the power of consciousness," which consists in our being alive. Your consciousness and my consciousness in that perspective are the same. At the same time, we each have a different mental structure that is associated with our consciousness. You are a psychoanalyst. You are German. You have completed a lengthy education. So it is not easy to separate these identities, such as "I am Hellfried, I have this education, I have this grandfather, I have children, I have a wife," from consciousness. The one is a subject, the other is an object. But they are so close! The Yogasūtra says they are so close that they appear to be one. That is what is called *asmitā*. *Dṛg-darśana-śaktyoḥ* is the quality of the mind. *Darśin* is that which helps us to perceive—for example, my memories, culture, religious background, or bank account details. Consciousness and the reality it perceives are different entities, but they are so close that they seem to be one. That means that things are different from that which is aware of them. This separation is difficult.

My cousin died. The moment life is gone, the person is no longer called "he" or "she." The word used is "it." It is a dead body. In our culture, a dead body has to be disposed of. Who is my cousin now? Is he the body or the one who died? Who is dead, the person or the body? That is the mystery. *Asmitā* comes from the Sanskrit word *asmi*, meaning "I am." I am somebody. I am that. I am this. The true "I" is different from the mind.

Anything that affects my body affects me; and what affects me affects my body. They say in Sanskrit it is like paper and what is written on it. They are separate, but they are also together. If I burn the paper, what is written here is lost. Before writing, nothing was there. The paper and what is written on it become one, but in fact, they remain different! You see my script on this paper. I cannot just easily wipe it off. This is what is called *asmitā*. So every change that happens in my system is for me a change that happens in me, even though real consciousness doesn't change.

We should also realize that we don't want to accept all changes that occur. For example, some people don't accept gray hair. Some eighty-year-olds dye their hair. They don't accept change. If I color my hair black, will I become a different person? What is growing old is not me but my physical body. The real me is timeless. It happens in relationships also. We have children. They grow up. They start to advise us. We cannot accept this, and it turns into a big fight because we cannot accept the change. So you are right, *asmitā* is a very strong factor in human life.

We can think of these *kleśas* like a tree. The root of suffering is *avidyā*, the trunk is *asmitā*, and the branches are *rāga*, *dveṣa*, and *abhiniveśa*. *Avidyā*, though we can't see it, is the dominant feature. You can cut the branches. Cutting the trunk is difficult because it is very strong. We never even talk about the roots of a tree!

H: I think it is also important, however, to recognize the role that the motivating factors *rāga* and *dveṣa* can have. They seem to be like fixed entities, something almost related to genetic influences. There may be people with a greater tendency to react with one or the other. Integrating these factors poses a big problem.

D: Yes.

H: *Asmitā* is the way I interact with my internal drives and external influences to build a unified entity from which I can say, "This is me." But how exactly do I do this? And if this is only the partial truth, how can I remove myself again from this state? Should we try to "dis-identify" again as far as possible? But then how are we to understand that all the things that bother me, and in the end cause me to suffer, are in fact merely identifications and not the truth?

D: The first step is recognition, not condemnation but recognition. This is very important.

H: Initially, I thought *asmitā* was something that in psychoanalysis we would call "narcissism." In psychoanalytic theory, narcissism means being self-centered, being in love with yourself, or egotism. Now I see that *asmitā* is a much broader concept. It encompasses any action I take while I am identified with it.

When I work with patients, I try to find out what they are identified with. I also investigate my own feelings and look at these feelings as indicators for potentially unconscious tendencies in the patient. If I am in a situation with a patient where I suddenly feel strongly that I have to support him or her, to be like a parent or give advice even though this does not appear necessary, I then ask myself what kind of role I have started to play for the patient. What kind of situation are we acting out together? What is the purpose of what I am trying to do with this person? I would try to understand all this as a part of the inner world of the patient. I would ask myself whether this situation could express my patient's unconscious desires and expectations of me. My identification with the desires of my patient allows me to attempt to form careful insights regarding my patient's inner world. I can then ask further questions, such as: Why should I play the role of a parent here? It is very possible that the patient tried to make me function like a mother because he was identified with a certain part of his childhood behavior. I can pursue this question and clarify it. Once these things are clear, it's as if a curtain has been lifted.

So you see, that which you call *asmitā* is an extensive process of mutual identification and a part of all psychoanalytic therapy.

I can give you a concrete example of how the analyst's unconscious identification with the patient's unconscious desires and experiences can be indicators of the patient's earlier relationships. I recently met a patient for the first time and was very impressed by his physical appearance. He had a strong, athletic body. I thought he would also have the strength to endure solid analytic work. For a long time, I was convinced of his robust nature. It was only after several years of analysis that I realized there was also a great weakness in his body. The patient also suffered from this false impression of his own physical strength. In this period of time, I used to go jogging. He somehow found out about this and decided to start running, too. However, he did this without any preparation. He was able to start running at full speed, and very quickly his pulse rose to 180 and more. I warned him about this, but he continued running. After a while, he began to feel unwell after running. I urged him to see a doctor, which he finally did. He went to see a doctor at the university, a very experienced professor, who also didn't initially believe the seriousness of the problem. He even joked, "With your body there won't be any problem." However, an examination revealed that the patient had two blocked arteries, which had to be cleared immediately by surgery.

This patient was the only child of a woman who was also a single parent. He had never met his father. His mother was fascinated by the athletic body of her young son, but she was unable to empathize with his inner state. All of us were fixed on the body. We were not able to look at his inner state, feel what was going on, and see the deeper part of his reality. Only after this medical procedure were we able to "dis-identify" from the idolization of the body. I think that I was, in his case, identified with the viewpoint of the mother.

So you see, not only can we therapists be identified with our own issues or experiences, which makes us unable to see reality clearly, but we can also become identified with issues from our patients or from their relationships. This makes matters very complex.

In psychoanalysis, we utilize this tendency toward identification in relationships to systematically examine problems in relationships. For example, when we conduct a supervision session with colleagues, we form a group and one member of the group reports on a problem he or she is having with a patient. As we listen, we try to discover what kind of identification this colleague has formed with his or her patient. If we are able to find out what this identification is, it is usually a great relief for both the analyst and the patient. The analyst is now able to see the patient with a new perspective, and he or she can disengage from the previous role identity.

That which you call *asmitā* is a central human phenomenon and has an impact on all parties in every relationship. In psychoanalysis, we learn to work with this phenomenon.

D: The first sutra, *atha yogānuśāsanam*, which I spoke about in the first chapter, can give us another clue. Here, *anu* shows that there is a continuous link between the student and the teacher. *Anu* means "I follow." The link that ensues is important. How can we recognize a person if we don't have a connection? Yoga is like surgery without the instruments. To perform an operation, you must touch the person, you must come into contact with that person. I cannot operate on the telephone. I have to be with the person. In surgery, something undesirable or some blockage is removed. In yoga, the term is *aśastra śastra cikitsā*, a transforming procedure without using external instruments. I need to *be* with the person, be linked with the person, for this to happen. This connection is what is often missing today in yoga. When I hear you say you have supervision and see clients twice a week, sometimes more often, it is clear that the connection is there. Unfortunately, I see that in the West, yoga often lacks this connection.

H: We could build groups where yoga teachers could learn this. That might be a first step.

D: This would create a feeling for the group as well as a community feeling. But when it comes to the personal encounter, how can one learn this in a group? We can't speak about everything in groups, so something would be missing. There should be training of yoga teachers who are also therapists, and therapists who are also yoga teachers at the same time. In this way, they could link up and come into closer contact.

H: Could we summarize by saying that relationship is very important in both yoga and psychoanalysis precisely because there will always be problems with identification? The yoga student as well as the therapy patient is always identified with a certain attitude or position. The teacher is also identified with something, even if it is just yoga theory or his or her own development as a yoga teacher. Within the context of a competent relationship, as described in the first chapter of the Yogasūtra, these attitudes can be reflected on, and if needed, they can be worked on as well.

D: In the fourth chapter of the Yogasūtra, it says: *nirmāṇa-cittāni asmitā-mātrāt.* This means: "If you want to reconstruct the mind from a negative situation to a positive one, what is required is a connection between the person who needs change and the person who can help facilitate this" (YS IV.4). We will speak about this in more detail later.

I would now like to further elaborate on *avidyā*. The fifth sutra in the second chapter discusses this:

> *anityāśuci-duḥkhānātmasu nitya-śuci-sukhātma-khyātir avidyā*
> Misapprehension leads to errors in comprehension of the character, origin, and effects of the objects perceived. (YS II.5)

Avidyā is when we are confused about basic things. For example, we consider something that is not going to last as if it were permanent. We think of something that gives us suffering as if it would give us happiness. Take addiction as an example. There we think that alcohol, drugs, gambling, or excessive food intake could make us happy, when in reality these things create dependency and suffering.

In India, we have the idea that certain things are clean and other things are unclean. Again, here there are many misunderstandings.

For example, in traditional times in India, when people belonging to the Brahmin caste went into a house that was not a Brahmin house, they then ate cow dung to recover their cleanliness. People could become ill from the cow dung!

There is also the concept that some things are not eternal and that other things are eternal. However, we don't know which. This is referred to by *anitya* and *nitya*. Our life is not eternal, but we wish it to be eternal. We therefore wonder whether other things that change are or aren't eternal. Instead, we should simply adapt to change.

In short, *avidyā* is present whenever our understanding of what we see and visualize is different from reality. This is not limited to just what the senses see; it could also apply to ideas and concepts. Patañjali's presentation of this is very open.

Śuci means something that is clean and *aśuci* something that is not clean. Our concepts of these are again affected by our culture and conditioning. For example, in earlier times, menstruating women were not allowed to enter the kitchen because they were considered unclean.

As you once said, we have certain set ideas, and we want to see everything based on these ideas. When we see something different, we don't accept it. For example, sometimes people cannot accept me as a teacher. Because I am not a typical "guru" with a beard and all those other Hindu accoutrements. They write to me and ask for an "audience." When they come and see me, they are shocked. "Is Desikachar here?" they ask, and I answer, "My name is Desikachar." They can't believe it. They are disappointed because what they find is different from what they expected. Their projection of a picture of me dominates their real perception in these cases.

Avidyā does not always occur to the same extent. That is a further mystery. Sometimes it is very strong, sometimes very weak. Sometimes it appears in one form, sometimes in another. There is this element of surprise because of the mind's tendency to fluctuate. It is therefore not easy to speculate on the exact quality of *avidyā*. It is not a horizontal line. It goes up and down. So you never know what will happen.

This fluctuation is because there are several states of mind. The mind may be quiet or agitated. Sometimes we are exposed to something and that provokes problems. Sometimes we have a craving and because of that something happens. In addition to that, things constantly change. I am not the same person I was when I was young. Many people cannot accept these changes. The Yogasūtra says that what you see might be real for you. But it is not real forever. Things change. *Sat* means "something exists." *Sat pariṇāma* means "things exist and things change," and we have to accept this.

How things change we don't know, but the truth of change itself has to be recognized. Somebody asked George H. W. Bush, "Is the president of America your son, or is he the president of America?" Bush replied, "When he is at my home he is my son, otherwise he is my president."

Avidyā occurs not only when we think that something that currently gives us unhappiness will bring happiness. The reverse is also true. Sometimes we think that something that gives us happiness will give us unhappiness. In other words, we can be mistaken in either direction. Sometimes we have to do certain painful things. For example, you are doing research. It is not easy. You have to do a lot of work to present a paper. So one of the aspects of *avidyā* is that something we think is going to give us pain is actually going to give us happiness. Something that will give us happiness now is later going to give us pain.

We have a Sanskrit word *moha*, which means "delusion." *Moha* is like a vehicle: you have a strong impulse to do something or get something, hoping it will give you power or happiness. We are almost blind and don't see the consequences. Sometimes *avidyā* can become *moha*. When the mind is not very stable, we have no control. Stability of the mind is very important in yoga but is difficult to maintain. There is a small fire in the mind. Add a drop of oil and the fire becomes bigger. A little more and it becomes bigger and bigger. The oil comes from outside. The fire is in the mind.

As a teacher, I meet many people. It's a challenge to know what my role is when somebody is in front of me. Suppose I am with a beautiful woman. Is my relation with the woman or with the person? All types of women come to see me, and I am a human being. Sometimes confusion about our life goals, our *dharma*, might arise. If I am busy looking at the beautiful woman and not the person, then there could be biological or emotional reactions. I could lose my connection as a teacher with my student. That would lead to bad consequences. Sometimes film stars come to see me. I don't know anything about film stars and am not looking at them as celebrities. I am looking with respect at the human being who wants help from me. As a teacher, I must always know what my role is, what my *dharma* is. I must be aware of this role and my relationship to the student.

As I said before, it is very easy for *citta* to become *manas*. *Citta* is something very close to pure consciousness. But this same *citta* can also become a slave to the senses. Then we are drawn in to the object and *citta* becomes *manas*. Recently, for example, I was invited for breakfast. I had already eaten fruit for my breakfast. We went to the buffet loaded with croissants, baked products, so many delicious things—forty items! I looked at the buffet and slowly the food started to tempt me: "Why don't you have me? It is for you. Anyway, you'll have to pay for the breakfast whether or not you eat it." In this way, my internal system was trying to justify eating. Fifteen minutes earlier, I had told those who had invited me that I would come along but not eat anything; I would just have some lime juice. But all this food was powerful and tempting. In the end, I didn't eat anything, but how tempting it was!

H: Where do we find this power to resist?

D: From a stable mind. Otherwise we can justify any temptation. The mind is powerful. The more milk you give a snake, the more poison it produces. We cannot reduce the poison by nourishing the snake!

H: In my view, sensuality and temptation are important parts of mental development. I think only people who are aware of temptation and who have struggled with it and even given in to it can develop the strength to withstand it in a healthy way. People who have not experienced sensuality are not able to develop this type of inner strength.

D: This is what the Yogasūtra also says. The idea that I have a stable mind and should not be tempted by anything is itself just a thought. Experience is what works. This is why the Yogasūtra says that if you want to develop detachment, to develop the mind, you must have experiences. Only through experience will things change. So you are absolutely right! It is only through experience that we can really learn something. That is why, in our tradition, you can become a monk only when you have first had a relationship with a woman and had children. Only then are you able to be a real monk and be called an *ācārya* (spiritual teacher).

Only one who has experienced and learned from that experience can tell another person, "I know what I am talking about." Transformation is not just an intention; it has to be achieved through experience, which sometimes involves suffering and effort. Only through *tapas* and *svādhyāya* can we achieve transformation that is profound, not superficial.

I recall a story about a friend. He went to the Himalayas for meditation. For six months, he meditated and felt he had reached the highest state of consciousness as a yogi. He had studied with me previously. After his experience in the Himalayas, he wanted me to see him. I agreed. At this time, I was teaching in an apartment. Opposite there was another apartment. A woman was living there, also a student of mine, who was working as a model. When he came out of my flat, this girl came in. He saw her for a moment. Three years later, he met me. He said, "I need a bigger house." "A bigger apartment for one person?" I asked. "No, not one person." He was living with the woman he had met during the lesson with me. She was thirty-two, he was twenty-two, but it didn't matter. They had two children, then divorced, then he married again and had four children, then divorced, married a third time, and had two more children. This illustrates that what one wants and what one does are often not enough to make these things reality.

I would now like to go on to the seventh sutra:

sukhānuśayī rāgaḥ
Excessive attachment is based on the assumption that it will contribute to everlasting happiness. (YS II.7)

Rāga is an emotional impulse that draws you to something in the hope of happiness. *Rāga* is the strong attraction of human beings to different things. There are three steps. We can imagine them like this:

1. Somebody says, "Oh, there is a place with fantastic ice cream. It is so tasty." Then I go there, and the moment I see it, I want to have it in my mouth.
2. Then I taste it and feel, "Oh! It is so delicious!"
3. Then I go home and remember the great experience, and I want more.

So *rāga* is experiencing, then recollecting, and then wishing to have more and more. It could be an ice cream or anything else. This could also include something that might be medically or socially risky. It doesn't matter for the individual involved at this point; *rāga* is so powerful.

The opposite is *dveṣa*. Instead of going forward and wanting to have something, here I want to avoid something.

duḥkhānuśayī dveṣaḥ
Unreasonable dislikes are usually the result of painful experiences in the past, connected with particular objects and situations. (YS II.8)

Dveṣa dominates when I don't want to eat something or don't want to see somebody, because of experiences I have had that feel unpleasant. Maybe I suffered some pain at a certain period of time. Now, fear of pain (*duḥkha*) discourages me.

Here is an example. When my wife went to Europe in 1970, she had a very bad experience. It was summer and this was the first time she was immersed in Western culture. Some relatives took her to the Saint-Tropez beach. My wife, a Brahmin woman, was totally shocked at what she saw there. Saint-Tropez is a nude beach. It was a horrible experience for her. My wife said, "I hate Europe. I will never go there again." The shock created deep revulsion in her.

H: Do you think that this includes certain kinds of fear? For example, when people are frightened to enter open places or when they avoid escalators or certain situations? This is what we call "phobia."

D: *Dveṣa* is the result of a bad experience. Fear, however, is related to danger—for example, the danger of losing your life. Danger is different from a bad experience, though they can sometimes function together. A friend had a bad experience at a hotel in Turkey. She was raped. Now every time when she goes to a hotel, she is frightened.

H: That was a traumatic experience.

D: Yes, this was a kind of trauma. Often we find combinations, multiple causes. This woman, for example, now hates men and is suspicious of them and thinks that they may harm her. She had to undergo psychotherapy to learn how to deal with this. Danger and fear are often linked to extreme situations involving life and death. Bad experiences, however, are something different. What my wife experienced was not dangerous; instead, this was linked to a deep-rooted desire to avoid something.

But as I mentioned, *dveṣa* and *abhiniveśa* often appear together. Let us now discuss this last branch of *avidyā*, *abhiniveśa*.

svararasa-vāhi viduṣo'pi samārūḍho'bhiniveśaḥ
Insecurity is the inborn feeling of anxiety about what is to come.
It affects both the ignorant and the wise. (YS II.9)

Why do we have fear? What are we fearful of? Fear is always there; it is inborn. Why does a child cry when it's born? Or we think it is crying. Is it trying to communicate? The Yogasūtra says, "The origin of fear is not linked to an object. It is inherent within us." Even a wise person is affected. The theory is that somehow, even when we are born, deep in the unconscious or somewhere, there is some anxiety concerning our survival. We see that with animals and with children.

Hindu philosophy says that in our previous lives we had an experience of death, where we lost everything. That threat of losing everything, including our life, is therefore contained somewhere in our consciousness or unconsciousness. That is why everybody has this anxiety or fear. Fear is linked to what could happen tomorrow. It could be death or any form of danger, and it is conditioned by past experiences. So Hindu philosophy says that in previous lives there might have been an experience of trauma or death.

H: Could one also say that that which Hinduism calls a previous life might also be experiences from the early period of a person's existence, when a person was still helpless? We can imagine, for example, a period in early development before a person has developed the ability of language. Vague memories could exist from the phase in life before one can speak.

D: That is exactly how I see it. Something may have happened. The child may have been alone for some time, or may have felt hungry and nobody was there to feed it. This insecurity could become the cause of the fear. Two aspects are present: desire for survival and fear of losing something.

H: What kind of loss is involved with this fear? Is it the loss of control or loss of the self? From the point of view of psychoanalysis, a child's fear of losing the mother is its greatest fear. When small children are separated from their mothers, they feel such indescribable fear that it's as if they were being destroyed. This point of view is speculative, of course.

D: Yes. We are in a mysterious realm here. We are so strongly linked to our body, our ego, and our position in society. We know theoretically that we are not meant to remain on this earth forever. Everybody knows this. Nonetheless, the wish for survival and our desires are very strong. I often wonder why people want to become billionaires. Some people are still pursuing this goal at the age of eighty!

H: In this context, they want to be loved and they want to be in control and to feel secure with regard to their survival. Take the example of a successful artist who has won every conceivable prize one could imagine. Nevertheless, he is plagued by sleeplessness and anxiety to the degree that his productivity as an artist is threatened. He suffers from a terrible fear of death. The thought that someone else could be a more talented artist than he is makes him feel as though his life were in danger. He feels he must be the best; otherwise he doesn't deserve to live. His continual desire for recognition, fame, and fortune is a necessity for survival. For him, there is some kind of anonymous force that could punish and destroy him, and he must continually earn his freedom by more and more success. However, if he enjoys too much success, he fears that jealousy from anonymous forces could also destroy him.

Only when he recognizes his own experience as the fatherless son of a psychologically unstable mother can he develop an understanding of himself. This allows him to understand his behavior and above all his faceless anxiety, as the fear of having an unstable mother, whom he must pacify and even control in order to survive psychologically. Processing these connections in the course of further therapy might allow this person to realize that he can alter his tendency to work in a ceaseless and dangerous manner, especially once he becomes aware that he himself has been a father for some time and is seen as a respected and model figure by others. In his anxiety, he had not been aware of this; we could say he had denied it.

In this example, we see the fear of death and compulsion to control in the context of an individual's experience, which can be understood if we analyze deeply enough. The important thing here is that understanding the causes can help us become free of the compulsive forces that drive certain actions. The fear of death itself remained, but it lost its compulsive and threatening dimension. Despite his advanced age, this person was still able to change significantly.

D: Now is the time to look at the fourth sutra of the second chapter, because it is the root of all the other *kleśas.*

> *avidyā kṣetram uttareṣāṁ prasupta-tanu-vicchinnodārāṇām*
> Misapprehension is the source of all the other obstacles. They need not appear simultaneously, and their impacts vary. Sometimes they are obscure and barely visible. At other times they are exposed and dominant. (YS II.4)

We have discussed the notion that we experience suffering because a structure within us called *avidyā* is active. It is like a color through which we see everything; that color is added to everything we perceive.

Recently, a yoga teacher from our school came to me and said that one of my students had had a serious allergic reaction. She had initially come to us because of back problems, and I had suggested massage and some breathing exercises for her. She had received massages for a few days before her allergic reaction, so I assumed that the massage oil had given her an allergic skin reaction. This, however, was *avidyā*. It turned out that after the massage she had used an aggressive, very strong soap that removes extra fat from the skin. So actually it was an allergic reaction not to the oil, but to the soap, which had removed the natural oil in the skin and made it excessively dry. I asked her to use a particular flower instead and soon she was all right.

H: In our profession, we would say this is a type of behavior where people unconsciously hurt themselves in some way.

D: Yes, but I did not say this to her.

So the sutra says that *avidyā* is like a field where many things grow. *Kṣetra* means "a field." Many things can grow on this field: wrong identification (*asmitā*); cravings or hoping something desirable will happen (*rāga*); displeasure, hatred, or anger because of bad experiences (*dveṣa*); and, of course, fear (*abhiniveśa*). And there are different stages. Sometimes everything is so clear, it's as if there were no *avidyā*, as if *avidyā* were sleeping. Sometimes there is just a sprout, not much, just a little. And then, because of circumstances or exposure to something outside, one factor becomes very strong. It could be *asmitā* or *dveṣa* or *rāga* or *abhiniveśa*. One, not all. If one is strong, the others do not appear. There is a metaphor for this. If somebody has four partners, he or she cannot be with all four at the same time. In a relationship, one can be with only one person at a time. Similarly, if one factor dominates, the others don't exist at that moment. So when one of the disturbances is very strong, for the moment the others do not exist. They may appear later. The source for all these confusions and disturbances is *avidyā*.

For example, I may dislike somebody, but I hear that person has some influence. He may help me to get a job. Then I will send some flowers to him. I will ask for an appointment, meet him, praise him, and try for the job. At this juncture, I will not talk about my dislike; perhaps it is not present at all. This happens in relationships, too. Sometimes we are unhappy with a person, but we have an interest in that person for other reasons. If that reason is compelling, *dveṣa* will not operate. We yield to *rāga*, and *dveṣa* goes away.

H: Does the factor that is strong represent the others, or are the other factors suppressed?

D: The metaphor I use presents *asmitā* as the trunk of the tree, with the three remaining *kleśas*—*rāga*, *dveṣa*, and *abhiniveśa*—as branches, so *asmitā* will always be there. "I love you, I hate you, I am afraid." The "I" of identification is always there.

H: So we can say that *avidyā* and *asmitā* are always present?

D: Yes. That is why the root is *avidyā*, the trunk is *asmitā*, and *rāga*, *dveṣa*, and *abhiniveśa* are the three branches, depending on the situation.

H: In our culture, we see hatred and love as being connected to each other, almost as if they were two sides of the same coin. Is this true for *rāga* and *dveṣa*?

D: I would say *rāga* is the first step for *dveṣa*. If there is *rāga*, soon there will be *dveṣa*, because at some point what is expected will not happen. In this respect, the two can be seen as two sides of the same coin.

H: When someone dies, for example, instead of mourning the death of their family member, relatives sometimes start arguing about the inheritance, even if there is not much to inherit or even if they are very rich. How can we explain this? Is *rāga* so powerful that it overturns all positive feelings? Or is something else behind this? Is it conceivable, for instance, that *rāga* or *dveṣa* serves to protect an individual from *abhiniveśa*, which may surface on the death of a close relative? I ask because we are speaking of the relationship between the *kleśas*.

D: I experienced something like this recently. Someone I know became very ill. He was sent to the hospital. It was a critical situation, and there were lots of tears. The relatives said, "We are going to lose this person who was so dear to us!" At the same time, they were talking about his wealth. Who is going to get the money? Tears were there and they were talking about money. Why were they crying, and for whom? Were they really crying for the person? If so, why were they concerned about wealth?

H: I think they do this to avoid being confronted with the reality of death and loss.

D: With all due respect, I feel greed and desire are very strong forces here. They start thinking, "Will I get the house, or will my son get the money?"

H: Maybe, but all this still covers up the experience of loss and death.

D: Often people fight over property after a death. They don't seem concerned about the person who died. So we have a duality: fear and sadness on one side and acquisitiveness on the other. This leads to confusion. The thought "What has he left for me?" becomes more important than "He is gone." I'm sad whenever I see this. *Rāga* is strong in these cases, which is why we say the most powerful emotion and force in the human system is desiring this and that. Some schools of philosophy believe this acquisitiveness to be even more powerful than consciousness. The third chapter of the Bhagavad Gītā mentions this.

H: As you said earlier, *abhiniveśa* is pervasive, deeply rooted in every animal system, and difficult to overcome. People constantly struggle with it. However, by focusing more on *rāga* and *dveṣa*, they may be able to avoid confronting *abhiniveśa*.

D: When my cousin died, his wife said, "Now I have nobody. What will happen to me? I will be all alone. I may fall, and there will be nobody to take care of me." That was her dominant feeling. Her husband died and her sadness was not really about his death. Then she added, "Oh, he was such a good person to me, he left this house for me, he took care of me," but that was not her primary feeling, which centered on her own insecurity. "I am all alone now because my husband is dead." Her blood pressure rose, she got palpitations, and a doctor had to examine her and give her injections. That is the power of *abhiniveśa*.

H: You see, the most frightening experience we as human beings can have is to be without any object or counterpart.

D: Yes.

H: So if there is *rāga* (greed, hunger, addiction), at least there is something to be oriented toward, or which you can grasp.

D: It becomes a very important diversion. I know someone who is seventy-eight years old. He had been married twice, and both of his wives had died. He then married a woman who was reasonably healthy and eighty-three years old, just because he did not want to be alone. It is not easy to be alone when you are old.

One of the problems we face is that we want to come out of our problems. We are willing to apply some effort. However, this effort can create more problems if we expect too much too soon. We cannot change the human system in one day! It takes time. This is why the concept of *Īśvara-praṇidhāna* is important. While you are putting out the effort, you must also have patience. When the river is flowing strongly in one direction, how can we change it to another direction? How can we stop it? It takes time.

Our desire for transformation and change may itself become a kind of *rāga*. And this is why many people become disappointed. My father once spoke with someone who had had asthma for thirty years. This person came to him and said, "Sir, I have been suffering from asthma for thirty years. I have asked all the doctors, but I still have my problems." My father said, "What do you want from me?" The person answered, "Can you please cure this?" My father replied, "You have had this problem for thirty years. If you can wait another thirty years, I can cure it."

How can you change a *saṁskāra* in one day? A thirty-year-old disease cannot be eliminated in one day. Someone might say, "I am suffering so much! I truly want to change," but one moment of lack of attention is enough to allow the old pattern to take over again.

H: It is important to emphasize the time required to change psychological processes. In modern medicine, there is now a tendency to address undesirable illnesses or developments quickly by surgery. For example, it is now possible for overweight people to use liposuction to remove excess fat and lose weight. These methods are sometimes unsafe.

Many people think it can be the same with psychotherapy. In fact, there are some so-called modern practitioners of psychotherapy who claim that psychotherapy should be completed within one or two weeks! We have to contend with these misconceptions about the amount of time needed to facilitate processes of change.

D: When people lose a limb, they often still feel it, even years later.

H: We call this "phantom pain." When applying this concept to obstacles, or *kleśas*, it means that the obstacles are not apparent as long as things are working as the person wants them to. However, the moment something doesn't work as expected, the obstacle emerges.

D: Yes, if they aren't visible, the *kleśas* are dormant. According to yoga philosophy, they cannot be destroyed.

H: How do we contend with this constant threat or danger?

D: We have to create another force so strong that the old force is rendered ineffective. That is what a later sutra talks about: creating a new *saṁskāra*. But this takes time.

Let us summarize some of the common points between yoga and psychoanalysis, some of the differences, and what they can both gain from interacting with each other.

The most common factor we have discovered is that the concept of relationship is crucial to the success of both yoga and psychotherapy. The difference is that in yoga, the relationship has to be established right at the beginning, while in psychotherapy the connection gets built up over a period of time. Another important difference is that in yoga, the relationship is always between a teacher and a student. In psychoanalysis, the analyst often has to take on a role—for instance, that of the mother or a support figure—to help the patient. It is important for yoga to reestablish an emphasis on connections and relationships—something that has been diluted, even lost, in recent years.

Furthermore, while yoga is very much aware of *saṁskāra*, or conditioning, it does not delve so deeply into life history. In therapy, the past is important, as it influences the present and the ways in which the patient acts. The past therefore has to be "brought up" and dealt with for the patient to improve.

Yoga has a strong notion of what can impede development: the five *kleśas* (obstacles) of *avidyā*, *asmitā*, *rāga*, *dveṣa*, and *abhiniveśa*. These concepts may be present in the West, too, but perhaps are not as clearly recognized as obstacles to progress.

There is also in yoga the central concept of pure consciousness: that which perceives other things and also perceives itself. In Western thought, this particular concept of active consciousness is not present; in Western understanding, consciousness is more akin to awareness or mindfulness.

Finally, the ultimate goal of yoga is inner growth. The goal of psychoanalysis is therapy and treatment. Both disciplines can learn a lot from each other, and in the future we can make attempts to train yoga teachers in psychotherapy and vice versa.

H: I think that there are concepts within psychoanalysis that focus on and deal with the obstacles (*kleśas*) in great detail. For example, greed (*rāga*) is a central concept in the work of Melanie Klein. We also assume that fear (*abhiniveśa*) is always present. In fact, the role of fear and uncertainty as a stimulus for our whole psychological development formed the basis of Sigmund Freud's psychoanalysis. Our identification with our environment (*asmitā*) is also seen as a basis for learning processes. We learn best from other people when we can identify with them. At the same time, we are aware of the danger of overly strong identification. The psychoanalyst Donald W. Winnicott has worked on this and developed sophisticated theories such as the concept of "the false self." A further aspect of *asmitā* is the feeling of self-esteem that feeds on identification with ideas and convictions. This area includes the theory of narcissism. Various schools, such as Heinz Kohut's psychoanalytic psychology of the self, have dealt primarily with this issue. So we can see that psychoanalysis works on phenomena similar to those of yoga, but the relationship is not the same and the method of approach is quite different. Psychoanalysis includes a whole range of different schools and theories, each of which places different concepts in the center.

However, there is indeed no concept such as the one you have described, of an active, self-perceiving consciousness, in Western schools of psychoanalysis. The closest thing we have is Sigmund Freud's comparison of consciousness with a light. But this is not a satisfactory explanation for the phenomenon that is central within yoga. On the other hand, it occurs to me that there are no mechanisms in yoga to reflect on the unconscious aspects of relationship. There must be reasons for this that are not yet clear in the context of our discussion. Perhaps we might say that yoga has focused more on pure consciousness, while psychoanalysis has focused more on the preconscious and the unconscious levels.

Both disciplines utilize the concept of relationship to work with another person in order to facilitate a process of development. This requires dealing with and overcoming forces of resistance. These forces are always present, as we have seen in this chapter.

In the language of yoga, these forces are the five obstacles called *kleśas*. In the language of psychoanalysis, these forces are seen as our unconscious resistance to change. If we seek to change, we must contend with these countering forces. As we saw in the first chapter, this works best if we are in a stable relationship with either a teacher or a psychoanalyst, depending on whether we are practicing yoga or undergoing psychoanalysis.

3

What Can We Achieve?

YOGASŪTRA, CHAPTER THREE (*vibhūti-pādaḥ*)

T.K.V. Desikachar: The third chapter of the Yogasūtra presents what we can achieve when we have established a strong and stable mind. For this, we need to put in effort. When we discussed the second chapter, we saw what kind of effort was needed. Once the mind is strong, many things can be achieved that were not possible before. For example, we can experience power, knowledge, and a further development of our whole personality.

The third chapter is called *vibhūti-pādaḥ* because it describes the great potential and the extraordinary power we have. It also tells us how we can achieve that power through meditation and introduces the various steps of meditation, the possible objects of focus, and how to choose this focus. It then reminds us that the mind is not always stable. Sometimes the mind is like a wave, which can at times be strong and at other times agitated. We therefore need some fine-tuning so that the mind will continue to be strong and stable. It also tells us something about the powers that may in fact disturb us. The point here is that we should not be tempted by these powers and shift our attention. We should go beyond them so that we attain inner freedom, not only for the sake of freedom itself, but also to avoid suffering.

Let us now look at the three steps of meditation:

- Step one is *dhāraṇā*, which is to fix a focus for your meditation practice.
- Step two is *dhyāna*, which is to remain with the chosen meditation focus.
- Step three is *samādhi*, which is to continue with this focus and go further.

Let me elaborate on what *samādhi* means. When the meditator persists with the chosen focus, the person meditating on an object and the object itself merge. A state is reached in which there is nothing more between them, and they become one. We can understand this more deeply by looking at the sutras. The first three sutras of the third chapter are as follows:

1. *deśa-bandhaś cittasya dhāraṇā*
2. *tatra pratyayaikatānatā dhyānam*
3. *tad evārtha-mātra-nirbhāsam svarūpa-śūnyam iva samādhiḥ*

So therefore:

- *Dhāraṇā* is to choose an object of meditation.
- *Dhyāna* is to enter into a relationship with this meditation object.
- *Samādhi* is to enter into an intense connection with this object.

Let us start with the first sutra in the third chapter:

deśa-bandhaś cittasya dhāraṇā
The mind has reached the ability to be directed [*dhāraṇā*] when direction toward a chosen object is possible in spite of many other potential objects within the reach of the individual. (YS III.1)

With meditation, it is very important to make the right choice of the object and then to stay with it. This needs preparation because it has consequences for us. We need to prepare the mental structure before doing meditation. In the second chapter of the Yogasūtra, Patañjali emphasizes that breathing is a very good foundation for meditation. The text says that attentive, extended breathing—*prāṇāyāma*—is conducive to making the mind ready for meditation. So, we follow the breath, then we regulate it, and we do this regulation consciously a certain number of times. The mind then becomes somewhat freer and can shed things from the past more easily. *Prāṇāyāma* is therefore an important tool for meditation. As the first chapter says, we must disconnect from something unfavorable before we can connect to something positive.

Hellfried Krusche: The third chapter talks about the development of special powers and abilities as the result of yoga practice. I would like to understand what this really means. Is it something that happens in the mind, in the realm of fantasy? Or is it something within the world of concrete reality? Are these abstract concepts or real powers and abilities?

D: That depends on the choice of focus. If I choose a tiger as my focus and meditate on it, I can acquire some qualities of a tiger. If I meditate on an elephant, I acquire certain qualities of an elephant. Similarly, when I stay in Germany for some time, I slowly begin to speak some German. This is all because of the process of association. We acquire certain qualities because of focused connections. We absorb qualities from these conscious connections.

The second aspect is one's potential. When you are depressed, you generally have less power. On the other hand, if your potential is good, you have more power. Let me give you an example. When younger, I was ignorant about health care and healing. I studied engineering. But because of my association with my father, I am now able to understand people who have health problems. Some things grow simply because of the environment we are in. When my daughter returned from America in August, she decided to become a yoga teacher. Now she is able to read pulses and has been able to learn things very quickly that she couldn't before.

H: Could we describe this process of connection as a kind of identification? The object is something I am connected with and am in contact with every day, and gradually I start to identify more and more with it. I become like this object. In some ways, it may be a sort of mimicry, but it seems also to be more than that. Through the process of identification, I can transform my personality into chosen aspects of the object. Would you agree with this interpretation?

D: Yes.

H: Imitation and identification are concepts in modern psychology as well. When your daughter sees you, she identifies herself with you, so she can learn more quickly than somebody else might. Is this a way to enter into an object at a deep level?

D: It is almost as if you become the object.

H: May I say that this merging is always linked to a person, to a personal relationship? I can understand this when you speak about identifying with people, especially in one's own environment. But when you say that this can also happen with abstract objects, it is far more difficult for me to follow. According to psychoanalysis, we cannot develop without a relationship to real people.

D: Here we come to visualization. For example, I knew a person who suffered from fear of speaking in public. I found out that he had great faith in the god Hanuman. Hanuman is a fearless monkey who was devoted to Lord Rama. I told this person, "Since you have faith in

Hanuman, meditate on Hanuman." I gave him a picture of Hanuman so he could visualize Hanuman and imagine him doing various things. Slowly he felt that he had received some blessings from Hanuman, and he began to have more confidence and less fear. So, when we visualize a statue or a painting of something in which we have enough faith, we can slowly create identification with that. This has happened to many people.

H: For this to happen, however, there must be faith and motivation and also the capacity to build this kind of relationship. In my experience, this is possible only if one has learned to develop stable relationships during childhood. There must be strong relationships, either between the teacher and the person or the parents and the person. In this example, there seems to have been a relationship to you that allowed the man to shift his devotion to an abstract object.

In psychoanalysis, we speak about the power of inner images, or about our relationship to our inner images. These inner pictures are the results of previous real relationships that have become established within our internal psychological structures and that can give us strength and assurance.

Where do you think this strength comes from?

D: People have so many gods. We are surrounded by gods. But often the choice is not made consciously. If the object of meditation is not selected freely, it does not have such an effect. But in some cases, as for this person who linked to Hanuman, it was chosen freely, not mechanically or according to what his parents said.

H: Psychoanalysis would say that this type of devotion to Hanuman is possible only if there have previously been solid, positive relationships.

D: Exactly. However, you still must choose the appropriate meditation focus. If this is done mechanically, it will have much less effect.

H: When it comes to a meditation practice, there must be someone who helps us make the right choice. There should be confidence in the person who helps us, and there must be *śraddhā*, the deep inner confidence and capacity to enable such a relationship. It always comes back to relationship.

D: We need a guide whom we can trust. The model is that of the teacher who knows the student, and the student who trusts what the teacher does. Whom can I trust? How can I trust? This is a big question.

H: A strong commitment is required here, one that has its roots within a stable relationship. But it's equally true that this process can be effective only if it originates from a place within the person; we could say that it has to come from the heart, so that impulses are oriented toward the right object at the right moment. Someone else needs to help sustain this, to support the student during this process. As we discussed, something in the individuals must enable them to build a profound relationship. I don't know if meditation can work without this ongoing support.

D: This is called "the faith factor." The Sanskrit term is *śraddhā*. When I trust the doctor, the medicine will be more effective. Faith in what I am doing is very important. *Śraddhā* is the most important factor in yoga. Meditation without *śraddhā* will not work.

H: What about the capacity to let go, to relinquish all effort?

D: Yes. This is very important. Sometimes when we are in a very close relationship, there is the risk of dependency. Our goal is freedom. Freedom means that we are not dependent on anyone.

H: Independent even of our own achievements? That would mean that the yogi should also be able to give up the influence, power, and money that he might have acquired? This reminds me of Shakespeare's play *The Tempest.* An Italian duke lost his fortune when his brother cheated him. He and his young daughter were sent out to sea in a small boat. Fortunately, they land on an island where he is able to resume his studies in magic. This gives him power to take revenge on his enemies. But later, when the duke gains control over his wicked brother and his brother's allies, he doesn't use this power. He gives them a shock and teaches them a lesson. He then decides to give up all his magical knowledge and power. It is an archetypal, classical, ancient concept: the powerful willingly decide to give up power.

D: My father had the ability to stop his heartbeat. When I asked him to teach me how to stop my heartbeat, he told me, "Don't learn such things. Do only those things which are good for society." He had this power himself, but he paid no attention to it.

I would like to elaborate on the three significant terms of the third chapter: *dhāraṇā*, *dhyāna*, and *samādhi.* Yoga speaks of meditation in three steps. The first is where I have many choices, but I am able to pick one. I choose this and not that not because it is attractive or beautiful, but because I think it will be good for me. It may not be easy, but with strength of mind it can be done, and in the long run it will be good. This is called *deśa-bandhaś cittasya dhāraṇā.*

H: So the choice is not made by the senses.

D: Correct. That is why the word *citta* is used and not the word *manas.* Usually the senses take over. Here, it is I who decide and not the senses. This is the first point. The second is, once I make a choice and begin to reflect on it, ideas appear, stemming from the object I chose from what I have been told and from experiences. It is like water beginning to flow, teaching me what is what. There is an interaction between what I see, input about that, and what is in my mind. There is an exchange from the mind to the object and from the object to the mind. This is interrelationship. The second step of meditation is an interrelationship where I give input and receive something. This process goes on continuously. This is all expressed in the second sutra of the third chapter:

> *tatra pratyayaikatānatā dhyānam*
> Then the mental activities form an uninterrupted flow only in relation to this object. (YS III.2)

When this happens, we may reach the third stage of meditation, *samādhi*. Suddenly, it is almost as if I am taken over by this great experience. I am not even aware of myself. I haven't had this experience before. The "I" stops; my I-feeling isn't there anymore. What exists is just the object I am focused on, at least for a few moments. This is *samādhi* as defined in the third sutra:

> *tad evārtha-mātra-nirbhāsam svarūpa-śūnyam iva samādhiḥ*
> Soon the individual is so much involved in the object that nothing except its comprehension is evident. It is as if the individual has lost his or her own identity. This is the complete integration with the object of understanding [*samādhi*]. (YS III.3)

Let us move to the next sutra, where *saṁyama* is suggested. Every day, my focus is the same. I have choices: for example, one day I can see the river, the next I can meditate on a beautiful flower. But this does not mean I am changing my focus. I have a particular focus, and it is always the same until I know everything about the object. This is something like scientific research. My focus, my interaction, and my total absorption is the same day after day. This is *saṁyama*, as the fourth sutra says:

> *trayam ekatra saṁyamaḥ*
> When these processes are continuously and exclusively applied to the same object, it is called *saṁyama*. (YS III.4)

When we have this continuous link, we discover new things. The clarity is absolute. We cannot predict when it will happen. It is like scientific discovery. As the fifth sutra says:

> *taj-jayāt prajñālokaḥ*
> *Saṁyama* on a chosen object leads to a comprehensive knowledge of the object in all its aspects. (YS III.5)

This is the essence of the first five sutras in the third chapter: *dhāraṇā*, *dhyāna*, *samādhi*, *saṁyama*.

Now I would like to move to the next sutra. Here we find the notion that we must proceed step by step. Our meditation should start from what is possible now, not from what our ideas or desires are. This is what the sutra says:

> *tasya bhūmiṣu viniyogaḥ*
> *Saṁyama* must be developed gradually. (YS III.6)

Our use of the tools of meditation must be according to our potential. If I want to study Freud, I'll have to start from scratch. You, Hellfried, wouldn't have to start there, but I would. What is possible for you in this case would not be possible for me. I would have to put in preliminary effort and after some time may come to your level. Similarly, if you want to learn certain nuances of chanting, you cannot do what I can, because I have been doing it for many years. That is what the sixth sutra says: We have to start from what is possible and then step by step go to our ideal. This is an important message. That is the attitude in which we teach meditation. First, we must know all the qualities, strengths, and weaknesses of the person. Then teaching can begin. If this method is not followed, there will be disappointment or disillusion. This is a very important point of Patañjali's. This is why in Indian culture in the past, meditation was taught privately and individually and consistently by one teacher. What was taught to one person was different from what was taught to another, for two reasons. One is the individual's qualities, and the other is their goals. As someone grows, we proceed to the next step and then the next, teaching something more interesting and useful. Timing is also crucial.

Meditation is not static; it is a dynamic process. This is another great contribution of yoga. The same thing is not taught to everybody in the same way; what is suitable for one person is perhaps not appropriate for another. Yoga individualizes the process.

H: I've always found it difficult to understand the third chapter. It appears that we have to choose a goal that is currently beyond our ability to imagine. I can't understand what exactly is meant by this. I understand that I have to choose an object, stay with it, and become one with it, merge with it. In the world that I know, however, people find it enormously difficult to stay with something and to connect so that they can merge with it. People as I observe them are trying to escape from such a situation or to avoid it completely. They are not trying to merge or to stay with a topic. In Western culture there might even be a fear of merging, because one then loses his or her individual identity.

If the goal of yoga is to allow this process of complete merging with an object, then I wonder how we can overcome the fears we have that are connected to this process. It seems that this is a process where one tries to come closer and closer to something one has chosen. But what is the real intention? When we try to come into contact with a God force, this is an intention; or when we try to alleviate our suffering. But what is the intention of meditation?

D: There are two paths in meditation. The first is to gain something. The other is to relinquish something. We could call these "addition" and "subtraction." In the previous chapter, we discussed the process of subtracting certain things to reduce suffering: for a person who is suffering, yoga practice can reduce suffering. A person with anxiety can use yoga practice to eliminate this fear. The third chapter is more about what I would call growth, power, and clarity. We have a model in India from the Bhagavad Gītā. In the Gītā, the teacher says, "People come to me for two reasons. They suffer and don't know how to resolve it, so they come to me for help. Some, however, want more than what they already have. They come to me and pray for more, for instance, for greater wealth." In terms of yoga, there are also two sides. There can be the wish to gain something and become stronger. Stronger not only in the physical sense, but in the sense of attaining the highest clarity, the greatest potential. In the first chapter, many techniques are taught to reduce mental disturbances: meditate on breathing, meditate on good company, pray to God, if you know someone who is a good adviser, go and listen to that person's advice. This is one track for meditation. The other is positive, in the sense of addition. Can I grow further? Can I become wiser? This is what the third chapter focuses on. If I suffer from anxiety and other problems, it is not possible to grow further. My first aim must be to reduce these fears and other obstacles so that the mind does not always worry.

It is not easy because we have so many problems. At the same time, we also have potential. The third chapter addresses this potential.

H: Does it deal with how we can develop this potential?

D: Yes. For example, Hellfried, before I met you I had a negative disposition toward Western psychology. I even said publicly that Western psychology spends too much time on the past and not enough on the future. I told my students: "Don't waste your time on the past. Think of the future." However, after getting to know you, exchanging thoughts, and meeting some others, I have learned something and have a better understanding of Western psychology. I have even encouraged many people to take advantage of it. I had been prejudiced against Western psychology, and you have altered that. Prejudice is a form of *dveṣa*.

People who have benefited from Western psychology have taken a step forward. I will never forget what you said once: "When there is too much ego, it is not possible to have trust or faith. Trust is vertical, ego is horizontal. Trust demands the ability to cultivate a sense of devotion or humility, and to be able to develop a vertically oriented relationship that can be invested with trust. As long as people suffer from an ego issue, they are focused on controlling their environment and therefore cannot have faith." That statement had power for me because I learned something. I have seen it at work. In India, although many people appear to have faith, their ego is often also strong. As a teacher, if I tell people what they are doing is wrong, they sometimes react by feeling hurt; they do not take it constructively. Some students get angry. They tell me that I am their teacher and that the teacher's role is to correct the student. But when I correct them, they get upset! Yet if I don't correct them, I am not doing my *dharma*.

H: In psychoanalysis, we assume that inner growth is a natural process and that it takes place when inner conflicts are reduced or solved. Our perspective is that a person experiences a dynamic process of development in relation to his or her environment. However, when it comes to developing something that has not existed previously, it's unclear to me how this can happen. I can imagine growth occurring from the removal of obstacles and the further development of something that already exists. I can't imagine this freedom of choice for a meditation object and the capacity that comes from the use of one's own will or power. We always see a person's ability to develop as coming from within his or her relationships to other people. It seems to me that what you are talking about is accessible only to people who are deeply rooted in yoga. From my perspective, this ability to merge with the object of meditation and experience something truly new seems impossible for a normal person who is engaged in everyday activities. I can imagine what you might mean by the term *saṁyama* only if I observe a scientist who has done research on a specific topic for a long time, or an artist. Here, I can see transformation of mind due to an ongoing, long-term activity. They become so identified with their profession that it is something like *saṁyama*, because they have done something over a long period of time and with deep commitment. We are approaching an area that seems mysterious to someone coming from a different culture. I could perhaps describe these processes by the laws of learning as understood within psychology. We learn by imitating and identifying with something, by proceeding step by step, and so on. But what is presented in the third chapter seems to me something more difficult to understand. It goes beyond these laws. I could even accept that the mind is something that changes continuously and that it is able to take on the form of an object. I can understand these theories on one level, but at the same time I can't really understand them. I can follow your words, but I can't really comprehend what you mean.

D: You see, first I studied physics and engineering and then I became a student of my father's. Today I am helping people with many different problems. My father told me years ago that I had to learn how to take a pulse. It was so boring for me, to take the pulse! He told me, however, to observe the pulse and that this would show me what kind of problem a person had. So out of respect for my teacher, I learned. It took me many years. Now I can understand people's problems by taking the pulse. I can't explain it, but I know it works. This pulse-patient thing has given me wisdom. There are some things that we must learn through our own experience over a long period of time.

Let's move on and talk about sutras 7 through 9 in the third chapter. Here the text says: "If the mind is disturbed, the whole system is disturbed. If the mind is quiet, the whole system is quiet." How did they know this? Nowadays it is scientifically proven, but how did they know this so long ago? For example, I meet a person, and one moment later I may meet a totally different person. The nose, eyes, and lips, the heart rate, the breathing, everything changes. The whole human system is of a particular structure. If the mind becomes agitated, the whole system becomes agitated. This is a very useful model.

H: Earlier you spoke about a person who underwent tremendous change after he established a yoga practice. May I say this change was possible only because he found a guide whom he could trust? Without this, he wouldn't have been the same. All the changes described in the third chapter—how is it possible to achieve such changes without a relationship or support or guidance?

D: There is a well-known saying that we can bring a horse to water, but we cannot force it to drink. This person you speak of decided, "I must do this. I must change fundamentally." I think the guide or teacher is one part, but the response of the person is even more important.

H: However, the sutras in the third chapter don't speak at all about the relationship between teacher and student.

D: Remember, the first sutra of the first chapter is: *atha yogānuśāsanam*.

H: Does that mean that this sutra is equally important as the other sutras?

D: Yes. We should never forget this sutra. It must be linked with all other sutras!

H: Can we reiterate what you said earlier? *Anuśāsanam* means "something that can be followed," and the sutra *atha yogānuśāsanam* means "to be in a relationship." Does this then mean that we should always keep the first sutra of chapter 1 in mind in order to understand the third chapter?

D: My father told me that when I meditate on the sutras, I should chant like this:

atha yogānuśāsanam yogaś citta-vṛtti-nirodhaḥ
atha yogānuśāsanam tadā draṣṭuḥ svarūpe'vasthānam
atha yogānuśāsanam vṛtti-sārūpyamitaratra . . .

Similarly, for the third chapter:

atha yogānuśāsanam deśa-bandhaś cittasya dhāraṇā
atha yogānuśāsanam tatra pratyayaikatānatā dhyānam
atha yogānuśāsanam tad evārtha-mātra-nirbhāsam svarūpa-śūnyam iva samādhiḥ . . .

H: So the secret in the third chapter, more so than ever, is that one has to always come back to the first sutra?

D: Never forget the first sutra. Now that I myself no longer have a teacher, when I have problems I try to visualize my connection with my teacher. I mentally talk to my teacher in a proper ambience. Sometimes I get a message. It is difficult to express how it happens. My father is dead. I visualize my connection with him. I had a strong connection with him. I am sure if he were alive, I would get an even better answer, but at least I get something. Wherever I am, I visualize my connection and something happens.

H: I have noticed that all the teachers at the Krishnamacharya Yoga Mandiram have a deep inner connection to yoga and are committed to what they are doing. This seems to give their teaching a special power and effectiveness.

D: Yes. But this is not enough. Both the personality of the teacher and the willingness of the student are equally important. It is like a chariot. There are two wheels. One is the connection with our teacher, the other is our effort.

H: And one doesn't work without the other?

D: Yes, exactly.

H: The idea that we must constantly keep the first sutra in mind seems to be essential if we want to understand the Yogasūtra. According to this, development in yoga is possible only within a relationship. The fact that this special dynamic can transpire only within a relationship, and that only then can the student acquire special abilities as a result, is a real discovery for me. Apparently, relationship in yoga is something that underlies everything else and as such is really the foundation. If I had merely read the sutras without your explanation, I would not have understood this idea. It occurs to me that this idea of a living relationship is not made clearly anywhere else. Books about yoga speak of the extraordinary powers and abilities one can develop as a result of yoga practice. Seldom does one seem to mention this living relationship to a teacher. Now I am able to see how *dhāraṇā*, *dhyāna*, *samādhi*, *saṁyama*, and the concept of *viniyoga* all become understandable as a result of a stable, long-lasting relationship. We have to reflect on the situation of the student and on his or her capacities and desires.

D: This is what is stated in the next sutra, the seventh sutra of the third chapter:

> *trayam antar-aṅgaṁ pūrvebhyaḥ*
> Compared with the first five components of yoga, the following three are related more to the inner world. (YS III.7)

Furthermore, the next sutra states:

> *tad api bahir-aṅgaṁ nirbījasya*
> The state where the mind has no impressions of any sort and nothing is beyond its reach is more intricate than the state of directing the mind toward an object. (YS III.8)

Sutra 6 in the third chapter describes *viniyoga* as *tasya bhūmiṣu viniyogaḥ*, as we already stated. This means that things must be taught according to the current level of a particular student. So things will be taught differently to different people, depending on what each is capable of. For instance, the object chosen for meditation practice can vary from person to person. For someone who has done a lot of meditation and practice, external objects might seem too obvious or coarse. This person may look for something more subtle, like an inner object. In sutra 7, this idea is further expanded. Here the text tells us to teach based on the inner situation and capacities of the subject. Sutras 6 through 9 develop the meaning of *viniyoga* in general. This is not a technique or a style; instead, it means to teach so that you can reach the student where he or she is now. When something is standardized, the real connection to the individual is lost. I already told you how meditation was taught in ancient times. The teacher had a connection with the student and had to find out the student's state of mind, abilities, and goals and how deeply committed the student was. The student had to be receptive and committed, but it was the teacher who had to find the right way to reach the student.

In our inner structure, everything is related. If I have never spoken German in my life and I say, "*Guten Morgen*," it is something special. However, after living in Germany, *Guten Morgen* might be nothing new, but giving a public speech in German would still be a big achievement. The message here is that we have to know the person's strengths and weaknesses. We need to comprehend what's possible in order to propose practice. With meditation, this is vital. We cannot standardize a particular method and teach it to everybody. Teaching you meditation by reciting "OM" would be silly because you would do it easily. It won't have an effect on you. But for some people who don't know "OM," it might be new and important to learn how to pronounce it and chant it correctly. This is what Patañjali says—that meditation should be taught respecting the individual's level of comprehension and current needs as well as his or her state of mind.

H: Can you give us a concrete example?

D: My father used to teach meditation differently to different people. For instance, a pregnant woman came to see my father. He said, "You are pregnant now, so you can't spend as much time on meditation as you did before. You may have nausea. Therefore, don't practice as you did previously, do it differently. Before you go to bed, meditate for only five minutes. Whom do you believe in? In the goddess Lakshmi? Then meditate on Lakshmi!"

When the baby was born and the mother was worried about the baby, my father would say, "Now you want your child to be healthy. Since you are focusing on the baby, whenever you feed the baby, mentally recite this: 'God, take care of my child. God, take care of my child.' " This is an example of *tasya bhūmiṣu viniyogaḥ*, meaning an appropriate adaptation according to the needs and current situation of the person. Life is like a wave going up and down. We have to teach according to different situations. One person decides to become a healer, and the teaching has to be changed to suit the growth of this person and his or her aspiration. Another person is in a temporary crisis because of family changes. Here we have to administer a simple practice, one that might have been too easy for this same person earlier. *Atha yogānuśāsanam* is the constant reminder. You must have a connection with the teacher from whom you want to learn. You should learn in a real interaction with a teacher who offers what is appropriate for the present moment: *bhūmiṣu viniyogaḥ*.

H: The concept of an appropriate connection plays a major role in psychoanalysis as well. For example, when we evaluate the efficiency of a psychotherapeutic treatment, we first look at the quality of the relationship between the analyst and the patient. We ask to what extent the patient has confidence in his or her therapist, and also to what extent the patient feels at ease with and understood by his or her therapist. It is expected that the analyst and the patient develop a common language, which means they both understand what they are talking about and can quickly and easily communicate. The ability to understand a patient and to communicate easily about the inner topics of the mind is essential for psychoanalysis. So once again, here we have some deep commonalities between yoga and psychoanalysis. This importance of an understanding relationship between someone seeking help and someone who can provide it seems to be a universal principle applicable in all cultures and essential for human development.

D: We say that when we teach meditation, only four ears should hear. Nobody else. That which is individual is also confidential.

H: Sometimes patients feel the need to tell their partners or friends what they have discussed in their sessions. In such cases, I feel we haven't yet found the right level of contact, that we are still building it. The real relationship starts when the patient stops talking openly about therapeutic discussions. Sometimes it may take many years before patients understand they have both the opportunity and the right to keep their inner lives to themselves.

D: That is what is meant by *anuśāsanam*. The student has to make up his or her mind to follow what the teacher says and to have confidence in that which the teacher says. This is how trust develops. The teacher must also be satisfied that a person can follow what is taught. That too is *anuśāsanam*.

That is why we need to test the student, to know if the student has real interest or merely casual curiosity. Sometimes people come to me for one day and ask me to teach them meditation. I tell them they have come to the wrong person. How can I teach meditation in one day? I have to know the student's background.

H: What about people who come regularly with trust and who are successful in their professional lives, but where it gradually becomes apparent that they have come only because I am useful in some way for their inner sense of balance? They don't come with the aim of finally becoming independent from me. It is as if I had become a part of their inner life. They tell me, for example, that I am the most important person in their life, that I know things that even their wives don't know. Sometimes I feel as though I have become a kind of assurance for their inner life. There is a long relationship, but no real contact. I feel as if I am a kind of medicine for them. Obviously they are motivated, they make some progress, but something is also missing. How can we understand this from the point of view of yoga?

D: This problem is very strong in our culture, too. I call it "dependency." It goes like this: "You are my teacher and you help me, so I become dependent on you. Any problem I have I put on to you. I come to you and you will tell me what to do." But this is not correct! The great thing about yoga is that we seek to become independent. From being dependent, we have to become independent.

The yoga teacher's role is to help the person to become independent. For example, this means "I know what the teacher has done; now I can take care of myself. Not only can I take care of myself, I can help others." This is the concept of *kaivalya*. "I am a free person and not dependent. I acknowledge and respect my teacher. But now there is light within me. Now that I have light myself, I don't need another person's light." That is the symbolism of *guru*. Literally, *guru* means one "who removes darkness and gives light." It is very important that the teacher ensures that we are not dependent on him or her, because that means lack of progress.

H: Yes, that is desirable. Nonetheless, it doesn't always happen. Some people say that they don't want to become dependent, so they don't come very frequently to therapy sessions. However, this can result in a situation in which someone will maintain this dependency precisely because the fear of dependence prevents the person from truly opening up to anyone. These people spend much of their lives avoiding relationships. They know many people, but they are not really connected to anyone, and they don't know why they feel so sad and so lonely despite the fact that they know so many people.

D: We should encourage all forms of independence. In India, there is indeed a great problem with dependency. We are slaves of our gurus and swamis. When the guru dies, the followers are shocked and cry like children. However, it should be the responsibility of a yoga teacher to help others so they can help themselves.

H: Sometimes in our profession we observe someone who resists doing enough to become independent. He or she will change just enough to stay in touch with the analyst. Such people create a situation where dependency is sustained. If they came three or four times a week for a certain period of time, we could work through the issues more easily and they would be able to develop further. However, they choose not to do this. Instead, they come once a week or every other week for many years, in a way that it is impossible to address a tendency toward dependency. It becomes a lifelong affair. In yoga, it may be similar with people who don't practice regularly and have issues they don't address and therefore cannot overcome. They decide unconsciously to remain dependent. You can find examples of this wherever gurus or therapists work with patients over a long period of time. What do you think about this?

D: You raise a very delicate question here! If someone comes to me, should I help so that this person becomes totally independent? If I succeed, I lose this person. On the other hand, there are also many others who could benefit from me. Should I confine myself to some, or should I be available to all those who need me? I tell people that they should apply some effort before they come to see me. I am there for them, but they must do something themselves as well.

H: Some people can feel powerful in life only as long as their guru or their therapist is in touch with them. This is the only way they feel sustained and empowered.

D: It's like teaching a child to swim. You cannot leave the child alone during the first swim. Slowly the child has to get used to the water. First we swim with the child, and later, we slowly reduce the floating aids. Then we can glide away in the water, saying, "You swim so well! Be careful."

H: I would like to add here that from the perspective of psychoanalysis, it is important to understand the fears that hinder people from choosing independence. Perhaps we need to look at these fears together.

However, it occurs to me now that we are discussing dependency when in fact the third chapter focuses on the special abilities and powers that can come from yoga. Why do you think this is?

D: This is because of the past. The past doesn't cease to exist just because I have a new connection. This is what the ninth sutra says. Sometimes we are in a state of attention and focus on something as if it were the only thing in the world. However, something from the past can take over, and then we are no longer in a state of meditation. It is like walking in the mountains when suddenly it starts to rain and get windy. I want a safe place. I find a small cave and go in. No rain, no wind, but I am wet and my clothes are drenched. The cave is warm, but I am shivering. That is an example of *saṁskāra*. It takes some time to let the "water" drip off and to gain some distance on what has happened.

This sutra explains that sometimes we are stable and sometimes we are agitated. Because of this, the past can sometimes dominate the future. Why?

The ninth sutra reads as follows:

> *vyutthāna-nirodha-saṁskārayor abhibhava-prādurbhāvau nirodha-kṣaṇa-cittānvayo nirodha-pariṇāmaḥ*
>
> The mind is capable of having two states based on two distinct tendencies. These are distraction and attention. However, at any

one moment, only one state prevails, and this state influences the individual's behavior, attitudes, and expressions. (YS III.9)

This sutra says that what happens in the mind will permeate every part of our system. If the mind is quiet, the whole system is quiet. The face, the breath, even the heart rate: everything will be stable. If the mind is agitated, the whole system is agitated. This link exists within the whole human system. This is a type of pattern, a *saṁskāra* that is like a habit or a condition.

However, it is possible to change things through effort. We can shift the mind from one level to another. That is the role of yoga. The purpose of the different aspects of yoga is to change the structure of the mind from an agitated state to a more stable state. If this happens, it takes place not only on an intellectual level, but as a complete evolution of the whole person. As they say, you know a Zen master is coming by the way he knocks on the door: The real Zen master knocks very lightly. The pretender will knock very loudly. He is not a real Zen master. The real Zen master is very gentle, very decent.

The real test to see whether something has changed as a result of a yoga practice is to see if the whole human structure has changed. This is apparent in many small ways: in the way in which I smile, how I look at you, and so on. This is described by the ninth sutra: every change in the mind will be reflected everywhere else in the system. There is a word that explains this: *pariṇāma*. It means "change." Our human structure is subject to constant change. The idea is that we can change that structure ourselves and that there are certain tools for this can give us hope. The sutra says there are three factors that help to facilitate change:

1. The first factor of change is nature itself. We have the potential to change within our own nature.
2. The second factor is time. Time is an essential element for change.

3. The third factor is our own contribution. The important thing is what we make of a situation.

Take someone who works with clay. If that person knows the properties of the clay, he or she can mold it into a beautiful sculpture. Another factor is time. If someone's nature is not open to change, then change isn't possible. This is what the next sutras say. So three factors are required to enable change: one's nature, time, and intelligence as a catalyst. Look at the example of a good farmer who waters the plants when needed, enabling them to grow. The bad farmer pours too much water at the wrong time and the plants do not grow. The correct application of water by the farmer is what I am calling intelligence. In Sanskrit, we call it *nimitta*. This is synonymous with experience. An experienced person knows what to do and what not to do.

H: What does "change" mean in this context?

D: It means that anything is possible. Change can go in one direction or in the opposite direction. It can be good or bad.

H: Can we also discuss what you mean by "nature"? Do you mean something like genetics or our early childhood and the way we have been raised by our parents?

D: Let us again take the example of clay. If the clay doesn't have certain properties, how can a figure be made out of it?

Another example: A scientist working with a certain material, for example, gold, has to understand the material's properties and possibilities. Clay has some properties that gold does not. Gold, on the other hand, conducts electrical current, but clay does not. It is these qualities that determine the kinds of change that are possible. I cannot make a mango grow like an apple, or vice versa. This is what is called "nature." This could be genetic; we call this *vāsanā*. This means something that has existed for some time before. I was trained as an engineer, for example, but I am not really good at it. I am good in theory, but not in practice. When it comes to repairing an engine, I can have an idea of what is required, but I am not a good technician. This is in my nature; we call this *svabhāva*. Sometimes this is dormant, and then, because of certain factors, it takes over.

H: As we just discussed, we should know the weaknesses and the potentialities of the person we are working with. The potential could be in the material constituents, as you mention here. From my perspective, there are many factors: vitality, genetic disposition, motivation, strength, energy, experiences, stability, and the capacity to enter into and to stay in a relationship. All these factors act together and result in the qualities of a certain person, or what you call nature. Would you agree?

D: Yes.

H: What about time? What role does time play when someone comes to see you for a consultation? Do you mean, for example, the person's age? Or the time he or she needs for change? The older the person is, the more difficult it may be to change.

D: Time is not the time of your wristwatch. We have to meditate on this. Time brings change. Our structure also changes itself. For example, there are some people I met when they were young whom I did not recognize when I met them again many years later. This is because of what has happened in their lives.

H: In psychoanalysis, we say that depending on the individual, the fast and major changes occur without external influence by the end of young adulthood, by the age of twenty-four to thirty. Development for older people occurs more slowly, meaning they need longer periods of time.

From our experience in psychoanalysis, we know that changes of the psyche need a long period of time. In general, psychoanalytic treatment takes three years before we reach a stable, lasting change. Treatment lasting longer than three to five years is not rare. Time has a big impact in our profession.

D: Sometimes change can happen to people who are past the age of fifty because of certain events or relationships.

H: You mentioned time, nature, and then something you called *nimitta*. What about love or other strong emotions as factors of change?

D: That again is *nimitta*.

H: So *nimitta* encompasses not only the event or a teacher, but also emotions?

D: *Nimitta* is like a catalyst. It is not simply intelligence, it is more. Certain things can happen in your life that open your eyes. Some events prompt us to reflect. Take my father. He was short-tempered and people were scared of him. In 1952, my elder brother, who was seventeen, could not put up with it anymore and left home. My father was sixty-four years old when my brother left. My father had great expectations of him. He was accomplished in Sanskrit and in yoga postures. But he could not put up with my father's temper. That transformed my father. From then on he was a different person.

H: He loved this son?

D: Yes, and he missed him very much. My brother never came back. Certain events in life can be a teacher. My father engaged in *svādhyāya*. He reviewed his life. People around him remarked, "He is now a tamed lion." After this, he had a lot of patience with me. He never lost his temper and never insisted on anything. Some events can be a very good teacher. Time is linked to these events.

H: But those events must have a strong emotional impact?

D: Surely. Some people won't learn otherwise. Of course, there are those who don't learn even then. I know someone who has had a lot of bad experiences and still won't learn. Maybe this is then a psychological problem.

H: If we say there must be an emotional event to trigger change, could we then say that such a person was emotionally closed up to this point?

D: Yes, and this is also a kind of arrogance.

H: Arrogance can be a way to protect oneself from emotions. In our view, there can also be a fear of emotions and a fear of losing control when feelings get too strong.

D: I will tell you a story about a person who was in the army. When he retired from the army, he became very cruel to his wife. She had to put on his shoes and socks for him. Sometimes he kicked her. One day she fell down and was seriously injured in the head. She had a kind of stroke that left her temporarily immobile. That taught him a great lesson. He repented, regretted his behavior, and from then on began to serve her. He is still taking care of her and has been doing so for the past seven years. He was transformed.

H: This event is also an example of *nimitta*?

D: Absolutely.

H: So the concept of *nimitta* is very wide. Any accident or a significant event that happens in life could also be a *nimitta*. It could be good or bad.

D: Once I was teaching a person meditation. Initially he did not take it seriously. Still, he came to me and said, "Can you teach me something to help me overcome some inner difficulties?" As he was a Christian, I told him I would like to teach him something in a church. I said, "Before I start with the next meditation lesson, let's go to the church." I took him to a very special church. I sat next to him and did some chanting. I don't know what happened. As I was chanting, he began to cry. He was fifty years old. For nearly an hour, he was in the church crying. Then he said, "I have decided to listen to you." Then I could teach him meditation. He is still doing it. He was transformed.

H: You mention this in connection with *nimitta*, the transforming factor. Can we say that *nimitta* is a powerful event that touches us emotionally in a profound way?

D: Yes, that is correct.

H: And *nimitta* may be different at various times and for different people?

D: Yes. It can be planned, but it can also happen like a sudden miracle. Let us now look at the tenth sutra in the third chapter:

> *tasya praśānta-vāhitā saṁskārāt*
> With constant and uninterrupted practice, the mind can remain in a state of attention for a long time. (YS III.10)

Change requires continuous effort. The more effort applied, the more change will be sustained. We can't do this casually. There has to be consistency in practice. The influence of the past is strong, so enormous, consistent effort is required to quiet the agitated mind and to keep it quiet.

H: This draws the emphasis to something new. Whereas in the earlier sutra we spoke about life events that have the power to change a person quickly, here we are focusing on continuity over a period of time. On the one hand, we have a shocking event that leads to a sudden realization, and on the other, a slow and continuous process over time.

D: Yes. Look at the army officer. Every time he sees his wife, it reminds him of what he did. Suppose she had died. He would have missed her, but I don't think he would be what he is now. Every day she is a constant reminder.

H: Would you say the event alone is not enough, and that it must be followed by steady application afterward?

D: Yes, exactly. The word *saṁskāra* has one more meaning, something like "to refine." We have to refine our efforts. We can't just function mechanically. The situation yesterday is not what it is today or what it will be six months from now. We constantly have to redefine the situation and refine our efforts. This is what I do with the people I work with. I don't give them a prescription for their whole life. That is why when people want help, I tell them I need to see them first.

H: In psychoanalysis, we try to adapt to our patients. We attempt to understand their language and to use this language with them. People have a tendency to hold on to old habits. They are used to engaging in relationships in an accustomed manner. They want to change; however, unconsciously there is something like a resistance to any actual change and to seeing their lives in a new light. Even the work with the analyst may become a part of this resistance. This can even happen to the extent that people come for therapy with the hidden purpose of not changing their life. They say, "I am in therapy, so I don't need to worry about anything else. After therapy everything will change." How do you view this?

D: Consider my daughter. She is still my daughter, but I treat her differently now that she is not a child anymore. She is developed, educated, she has transformed herself, she is attentive. The way I communicate with her today is not the way I communicated with her two years ago. I see her now as my equal.

We have to see where the person is now to decide what we should do. This is refinement. We constantly have to refine our techniques to adapt to the present situation to enable continuous growth. Otherwise, we may even regress. It's amazing how people knew this in ancient times.

H: That means that depth of contact and closeness to the student inevitably lead to development. This is indeed ancient wisdom! It also fits well with modern psychoanalytic treatment, which came into being two thousand years after yoga. In many psychoanalytic schools, for instance, the quality of the exchange and the closeness of the relationship between the patient and the analyst are the most important aspects of treatment. Here the movement of the patient from one state of mind to another state of mind is meticulously observed and analyzed in every session. We also have the understanding that the mind is constantly moving from a state of clarity and focus (or as you would say, from *citta*) to a state of entanglement, fear, and lack of clarity (*manas*). It truly oscillates between both of these states. The first state is an integrated, stable position, whereas the other state is one where fear dominates. The same person can move from a fearful state to a calm state in different situations, and vice versa. The job of the analyst is to see this, to follow it, and to respond according to the patient's current situation. So in psychoanalysis, we also see the mind as something constantly shifting, which has to be followed if we want to stay in contact with it. Some psychoanalysts now say that we can contribute to a patient's inner growth only to the extent that we are able to follow the patient's mental movements. If we are able to move with them, the patient can more easily overcome internal resistance to change and hence develop.

However, we psychoanalysts don't have a simple and direct concept of growth as you do in yoga. In our profession, we see growth as taking place when we are able to remove obstacles and develop a close and stable relationship to the patient. So we are more concerned about working through and removing obstacles. It seems to me yoga is oriented more toward active growth and development of the person. The goals of growth are also clearly defined in yoga: the primary objectives are inner freedom and achieving states, or abilities, that were not previously possible.

4

How Can We Gain Inner Freedom?

YOGASŪTRA, CHAPTER FOUR (*kaivalya-pādaḥ*)

T.K.V. Desikachar: The fourth chapter of the Yogasūtra is especially important for people who work with the mind. It deals with the question: How can a person transform? And the main focus of the chapter is: What is change?

Change, or transformation, in the context of yoga means:

- A person who was previously unable to do something can now do it.
- A person grows to comprehend things he or she could not before.
- Someone previously unable to develop further can now develop.
- Someone who was unable to engage in a deeper relationship with another person because of things that happened in the past can now have this kind of connection with someone.

How is this possible? How and on what basis can such developments occur?

The first sutra in the fourth chapter tells us that transformation is sparked by a variety of factors:

> *janmauṣadhi-mantra-tapaḥ-samādhi-jāḥ siddhayaḥ*
> Exceptional mental capabilities may be achieved through genetic inheritance, the use of herbs as prescribed in the sacred texts, recitation of incantations, rigorous austerities, and that state of mind that remains one with its object without distractions. (YS IV.1)

The factors mentioned in this sutra are as follows:

1. *janma*
2. *oṣadhi*
3. *mantra*
4. *tapas*
5. *samādhi*

Janma means that something that was hidden suddenly appears. For example, in the springtime all the trees and plants suddenly start to grow again. Something suddenly manifests itself because the potential was there. That is what *janma* means: some people have potential within them, and without applying effort at some moment this appears. Great musicians, prodigies such as Yehudi Menuhin, are examples of this. Menuhin could play music at a young age even without a teacher. This is *janma*. It is inborn, an inherent quality. There is no need to exert effort; slowly or suddenly it presents itself.

On to the next term: *oṣadhi*. This refers to substances such as herbs and drugs. In India, in the past many people believed that certain leaves and flowers had special effects. If you used them in a ritual and offered them to a higher force, and then ingested the remains, it was believed that your mind would be transformed. We have ancient rituals in which certain leaves called *soma* are used. A particular ritual performed to produce these remains was called *soma-*

yagya. The people who performed these rites believed that the remains were coming directly from a godly force. They also believed that consuming them would lead to significant change. There's an Indian myth that symbolizes this: The demons and gods were churning the ocean. They churned and churned and churned. Suddenly something started to form from all this churning. This was called *amṛta* and it was believed that if you took a drop of it, you would become immortal. A drop of this *amṛta* was all you needed to become an immortal being. You wouldn't have to apply any effort, just ingest a drop of this.

Modern medicine has developed many substances that can change our system. Psychiatrists, for example, administer medications for depression or other illnesses. This could also be called *oṣadhi*.

Now we come to the term *mantra*. When a teacher has done a lot of meditation on a certain mantra, he or she is in a position to give this mantra to the student. The student will then use this mantra exactly as it was taught by the teacher. Belief and faith in the mantra can then impart certain qualities that were not there before. In India, this is common. For example, a friend of mine who had no self-confidence was invited to give some public lectures. She came to me for help. I asked her if she had faith in Hanuman. Hanuman is a very well-known, powerful god in India. "Yes," she replied. So I taught her how to meditate on Hanuman using a particular mantra on Hanuman. I asked her to recite this mantra every day for forty days and then to decide what to do. I also instructed her to visualize and think about Hanuman, who was so courageous and had no fear, when reciting the mantra. Forty days later, she came back and said, "Somehow I feel that Hanuman is taking care of me." She gave her presentation and everybody admired her. Some of her friends even asked, "How did you do that? Where did you find such courage?"

Reciting a mantra can endow us with qualities that the mantra represents. When we apply effort over time, the qualities of the mantra are imparted to us. In the first chapter of the Yogasūtra, Patañjali says, for example, that if you visualize *Īśvara* and then you recite the *praṇava* (OM), your obstacles will be removed and you will discover yourself.

The next point is *tapas*. This refers to a technique that reduces inner impurities. There's a reference to *tapas* in the second chapter of the Yogasūtra, in sutras 1 and 43. If there are impurities in the mind, in the senses, or in the body, then the term *tapas* refers to practices that can reduce these impurities. *Prāṇāyāma* (the conscious breathing discussed in chapter 3) is one of the most important *tapas*. *Tapas* should be applied in a careful manner. This is very important! Sometimes people try to do too much. *Tapas* should be practiced in a way that it does not disturb the mind—otherwise it is not *tapas*. For example, some people do too much and then lose their temper or their nerves or the ability to communicate with others. More than two thousand years ago, Patañjali said *tapas* must not disturb the mind and it should be done respecting our limits and our resources. *Tapas* is also linked to diet. The right type of food consumed in moderation is another aspect of *tapas*.

The last factor named in this sutra is *samādhi*. Here the word *samādhi* refers to the complete system of *aṣṭāṅga yoga* and is identified as the best method to achieve certain desirable qualities. So *samādhi* in this sense includes the social relationships of *yama* (our behavior and attitudes toward our environment) and *niyama* (our behavior and attitudes toward ourselves), as well as *āsana* (physical postures), *prāṇāyāma* (breathing exercises), and the three steps of meditation. Here the order of listing all the various factors is significant, and the last in the sequence is the highest or most important. That is why *samādhi* is called the fifth and final factor and is considered the best method. The person who has been transformed through the *aṣṭāṅga yoga of yama*, *niyama*, *āsana*, *prāṇāyāma*, *pratyāhāra*, *dhāraṇā*, *dhyāna*, and *samādhi* is the true teacher.

Hellfried Krusche: The sutra first mentions *janma*, which is an innate, inner quality one is born with. We do not have to do anything actively. Patañjali then continues with *oṣadhi*, a medicine or drug, which we only have to ingest. With *mantra*, for the first time we have to apply some effort. For *tapas* and *samādhi*, we have to apply discipline and practice in an even more active way. Interestingly, you said that the last (and hence most important) factor mentioned is *samādhi*, which includes here ways of relating to the external world (*yama*) and the internal world (*niyama*). In yoga, both discipline and the manner in which we relate to our external and internal worlds are of key importance.

D: There is a difference between a guru and an *ācārya*. *Samādhi* is the process an *ācārya* goes through. *Janma* and all the other factors lead to becoming a guru. That is why some people who are prodigies, extremely talented in some area, are not necessarily very good teachers. If they are not disciplined, they cannot identify with the problems that other, less talented people have.

We had a flute player in India who was marvelous. Even when he was drunk he was great. However, he was not able to teach others to play. He performed well and earned some money. Slowly he started to drink more and became addicted to alcohol. In the end, he could barely give concerts. Nobody could play the way he could play, but he became a disappointment. This is from his birth, *janma*.

On the other hand, those who have learned music know about high notes and low notes, because they had to apply a lot of effort. That is *samādhi*: effort and discipline. People who have followed this path are considered *ācārya*.

H: May I add that *samādhi* again underlines the important aspect of relationship?

D: Yes, it's good you raise this point again. It is important that one does not simply follow or develop a habit; there must also be a sustained relationship involved. For example, with *mantra*, the guru may simply give a person a mantra and then there is no connection anymore. With yoga, on the other hand, we have a steady relationship between teacher and student. The teacher watches and guides just as a mother guides her child when it is born, step by step, until she is able to let the child go. This is not a random or temporary connection, but a sustained relationship that can transform the student.

H: So at the center of yoga instruction is the idea of development within a sustained and reliable relationship?

D: Yes, and this doesn't happen in one day. It requires a lot of patience. When I learned Vedic chanting from my father, I admired his patience toward me. He was a great chanter and a great musician. I, however, was not a good singer. I also wasn't able to listen very carefully. My father was so patient with me. My mother, on the other hand, used to say, "Why are you trying to learn chanting at this age? It is not even necessary." I was touched by my father's patience. I never missed a lesson with him. He never criticized me, though I made a lot of mistakes. Whenever I teach people, I remember how patient my father was. He knew so much. He could have said, "You are unfit for chanting, give it up." He never said that. I knew so little, yet he managed to have patience with me, and I have therefore learned to have patience with my students. So that connection has been a good reminder for me.

The first sutras emphasize that we all have potential. It is not that we get it from somebody else or that the teacher gives us something. We have potential, and depending on our good fortune or our good relationships or our own good efforts, our potentials may grow.

I have a question for you. Sometimes I've seen people who practice *āsana*, *prāṇāyāma*, and meditation, but nothing happens. There is no transformation, no change in the person. They know all the texts, but there is no transformation. I've also seen people who have spent very little time with such things but nonetheless have really been transformed inside. How can we understand this?

H: From the perspective of psychoanalysis, I would say this depends on the quality of the relationships a person had in childhood. Experiences of relationships with people who are emotionally important to us can transform into inner structures of our psyche. We call the result an "inner object." In psychoanalysis, we see people as being in relationships not only with external objects, but also with these internal objects. Internal objects are our experiences and images that we have developed out of our early relationships and experiences with other people. They are also the inner images of our reactions to certain important events in our lives. If we have had helpful, positive experiences in both our internal and external worlds, then we are more likely to be open to opportunities to develop and transform ourselves in the future. However, if we have so-called negative objects in our internal and external worlds, then we tend to experience our environment as threatening and controlling, and we are then more likely to react to opportunities for change in a defensive or withdrawn manner instead. We are not as able to learn and develop because we are primarily involved with protecting ourselves.

The capacity of a person to be involved in positive relationships with other people increases the chances that he or she will be open to further development. If someone's yoga practice is a mechanical repetition of exercises and there is no relationship with his or her teacher, then he or she may develop technical abilities, but mental structures won't be changed as a result of this practice, because the person's relationship experience will not be connected with yoga. If we truly want to change, then we must enter into a relationship with a person important to us who can truly touch us. If this is possible with the yoga teacher, for example, then a transformation is possible.

Sometimes I also meet people who engage in yoga or psychotherapy without managing to change anything fundamental in themselves. These people are apparently able to do these practices mechanically without letting transformation happen. In fact, it is not uncommon for some people to use yoga or psychotherapy as a way to avoid change. The impetus lies within the person and comes from the inner world in which he or she lives. Some people who receive relatively little help can change tremendously. These people have developed an inner world with positive or helpful internal objects. They form an attitude that is open to relationships and does not see them as threatening. They therefore have less fear of change and can more easily take on suggestions from a teacher or therapist.

The ability to change and grow varies from person to person, and other factors are involved—for example, genetic influences. Within psychoanalysis, we focus predominantly on the aspect of relationship.

D: Some people say that they put their faith in God. They may donate money, pray, or perform certain actions. I sometimes observe these people when performing a ritual, and it is almost as if they are wearing a mask when they enter the temple. Afterward, once the ritual is completed, they return to being a different person. They believe religion is one thing and life is another. And that having a relationship with a person is little compared a relationship with God. How is it possible that they aren't available to change?

H: I see this as a splitting of the mind. There are at least two aspects to your question. First, there is the structure of the specific personality; then there is the question of religion. Human psychic structures are complicated; we must always take this into account. It could be that a person has several states of mind, or let us say split layers of the personality, without the person knowing it. We call this "splitting of the mind." In severe cases, this can lead to psychotic behavior. In fact, many people have different, disconnected parts in their mind, and one part doesn't know what the other part is doing or thinking.

D: Like Dr. Jekyll and Mr. Hyde?

H: Exactly! This famous story clearly demonstrates this phenomenon. You often find this split structure with people addicted to alcohol or other drugs. But in a less pronounced form, you can find it in apparently quite normal people. A man may be cruel and terrifying at work, whereas at home he may be an attentive father and even a subservient husband. Splitting of the mind is a strange psychic phenomenon, but also a typical human trait. The layers of consciousness of people suffering from this phenomenon are often divided out of fear of losing control over their environment and over themselves. If we want someone to reduce splitting his or her psyche, then we need to work with that person to address his or her fears. Understandably, change to that person represents danger or sometimes even catastrophe. This may mean that we need to do longer-term work until the person becomes more "united" inside. This kind of work is not easy and requires time and patience, but it is possible to achieve. Then that person too can truly transform.

Regarding the second part of your question: When it comes to religious feeling, I can't answer from the theoretical field of psychoanalysis. Our theories do not have much to say on this topic, and there are great differences of opinion among my colleagues. My own opinion is that experienced religiousness is also about relationship. However, the nature of this relationship is different: it is something I call a "vertical relationship," meaning a relationship to something higher. You can't be taught to have this. You have to feel and experience it. Psychoanalytic work can help develop this kind of attitude insofar as it helps a person free him- or herself from old, debilitating internal conflicts—in other words, freeing the inner world from unconscious conflicts. The result of this freedom should be that the structure of the personality becomes unified and not two or more split aspects of a personality. Psychoanalytic work involves penetrating those compartments and dissolving split aspects into a whole psyche. My own view is that a person who is able to resolve his or her fears and who can experience him- or herself as one personality has a greater chance of becoming an authentically religious person. I also believe that meditation requires healthy mental functioning. Otherwise, there's a serious danger of developing psychological illnesses and becoming mentally stuck.

Let's take the example of a patient who came to me because he could no longer meditate. For many years, he had been accustomed to sitting for thirty to sixty minutes in the morning in a silent Zen meditation. Recently, he had become unable to sit in meditation because of agonizing thoughts. He had also lost the ability to connect to that which he called "God." He sought help from a clergyman, who sent him to me.

Over the course of what turned into a lengthy treatment, it came out that he had an eating disorder. We were able to determine that this eating disorder stemmed from the fact that his mother left him when he was a small child. Disappointment at being abandoned by someone important repeated itself a number of times in his life. Although he was a fun-loving person, he had become quite lonely and bitter and had lost all his friends. When he came home alone at night and started to eat, he could not stop. He had to stuff himself completely. He became fat, stodgy, and reclusive.

Unconsciously, he had repeatedly re-created the situation of being abandoned, as if he needed to relive being a hungry, deserted child. This had led him slowly to hate other people, and this hatred was what prevented him from finding peace in meditation.

In his ongoing work with me, which lasted over several years, he was able to look at his deep wounds and to learn to speak about them. Only after the connections between these factors had become clear and he was able to feel them could he start to give his life a new direction. He met a girlfriend who was very good for him. He no longer felt so lonely and helpless, so food became less important and he was able to lose weight.

Ultimately, he came to understand that he had practiced meditation in a way that maintained his loneliness: he had chosen a practice in which one remains for days without any contact with other people, and his connection with his meditation teacher was infrequent and superficial.

This example demonstrates how meditation without real direction can become a part of an illness. Luckily, this particular patient was strong and motivated enough to escape from his predicament. In extreme cases, and with people who are not as stable, psychological illness can develop in the place of religious feeling. We always work on deepening the capacity of the person to be in a relationship. This also means having a balanced relationship toward oneself, and that implies the ability to have empathy for others without losing the ability to feel whole oneself. This is why it takes time to treat these kinds of problems. You once said you need to see a person in different situations if you want to get to know him or her. Similarly, we also need to get to know a person before we treat him or her, and this involves the dimension not of space but of time. We want to see a person in different time periods over the course of his or her life.

D: My father spoke about a difference between *ayoga*, *yoga*, and *yoga-yoga*. He said people who practice yoga as if it were a technique do *ayoga*, which is not really yoga at all. On the other hand, those who are connected with something else are doing *yogayoga*. For him, yoga was connection.

The second sutra in the fourth chapter explains how changes happen, according to the perspective of the Yogasūtra:

> *jāty-antara-pariṇāmaḥ prakṛty-āpūrāt*
> Change from one set of characteristics to another is essentially an adjustment of the basic qualities of matter. (YS IV.2)

The fascinating idea being presented here is that everything already exists. For example, in the ground outside this window there is water, there is earth, there are roots. We might not see the water, but this does not mean there is no water. Suppose we dig a little, then we will find water. If we dig into the soil, we will also find roots. This is what the sutra says: We already have everything; however, not everything is manifest. When certain things suddenly surface in your inner world, you can appear to have become a different person. That is what is called *jāti*. *Jāti* means that something that was hidden now appears. It comes from the ancient word *jani*, which loosely means "everything is already there." If that which was previously hidden is revealed, then the person is no longer the same. The next sutra says something about the actual mechanics of how this works. So the second sutra says that all the abilities we have are there not because something external gave them to us. Instead, it says they were always there in us and they can suddenly appear because of certain changes.

Here's a simple example. Two years ago, my daughter gave me a pen as a gift. About six months ago, I couldn't find the pen. So I told my daughter, "I am so sorry that I don't know where it is—I cannot find the pen. But I am very confident that one day I will find it! I don't know where it is now, but it will turn up." For six months the pen was missing, and then one day my wife found the pen in the bed when she was changing the mattress. I had been sleeping with the pen under my mattress, but I never found it. When the mattress was changed, there it was.

This example also illustrates a difference between yoga and Hinduism. In the Hindu religion, there is a belief that God gives you everything and that is why you have it. You did not have it before, but now God gives it to you and then you will have it for the first time. The Yogasūtra takes a different position. They say that everything exists, but some things do not appear, which means simply that they are not activated. However, change can facilitate their appearance. The yogic principle is, everything exists and everything changes. When the sun sets, the sun is not gone. It will reappear. What do you think about this idea?

H: In the traditional Western concept of learning, learning something new means to bring something new inside of you. In other words, learning means something external is added to the system.

But the worldview you describe here is very different. Instead of adding something new, one uncovers what is already there. As a teacher, you try to create circumstances in which an individual may develop something new by letting what is within him or her come to the surface. This is a completely different way of looking at people and learning. If we take this view, then rather than trying to give people something that may or may not be appropriate for them and that they may not even want, we should create optimal learning environments instead. One should try to help people overcome old habits and discover what is hidden within them. So it is a matter not of putting something into a person, like into a machine, but of creating situations where a person has a chance to develop. This seems like a humanistic view of the world, and one I can readily agree with.

When looking at people this way, we cannot be quick to judge them. Instead we must endeavor to look deeper, to see and understand them in the context of their total situation before we can say anything. We cannot say someone is crazy if he or she acts in a bizarre way; we would say that in this particular moment, he or she has a particular problem because of certain momentary forces.

D: Exactly. The factor that leads to the change is what you would call dormant.

H: Some psychoanalysts say that we have to follow a person in every mental state he or she may be in during treatment. Patients may be in completely different states of mind from one session to the next. Sometimes they may be considerate, friendly, and calm; the next time they can be driven by hatred or extreme anger. Their attitude toward the therapist can also change: they might see their therapist during one session as a friend or helper, then perceive the therapist to be a danger or enemy. Patients may also exhibit changing states of consciousness. Sometimes they may appear a bit crazy, the next session they seem calm and clear, then later they appear depressed. We try to follow patients in their changing states of mind and to be present during these changes and to the shifts among the various states of consciousness. If we can manage to do this, we are often able to impart a sense of continuity and safety to patients. They come to realize that among all the changing states of mind, there is one consistent factor and that is the stable, safe foundation in relationship. We believe that people carry this knowledge within them, but often they forget this in the course of their lives. During treatment, we endeavor to remind them of this.

D: The Gāyatri mantra, which we recite every morning, is an example of the idea in this sutra. We sing, for example, "Sun, we praise you. Take away our impurities. We meditate on you. When we meditate on you and your great clarity, then our clarity is revealed, and our courage is renewed." This does not mean that the sun gives us clarity. It is more that the sun allows the clouds, which dampen our own clarity, to be removed so the light of our own clarity can emerge. Clarity is always here inside us; sometimes clouds or other factors dampen or block our meditation and our light. Then we use certain tools to address this. It is like a garden; something is always changing!

H: We are given a picture of continuity, of a supportive background that despite ongoing change remains stable and conducive to clarity. This makes me realize how difficult it is to give someone advice. How is it possible, when you never know what the outcome will be? How do you know what you should do to help someone? Perhaps the only thing we really can do is to be present for the person and to create an environment favorable to his or her development?

D: Yes. For example, suppose you want to learn how to surf. You go to the ocean and look at the conditions. You have to examine the water to see if the waves are good and how the tide is, and based on this you will decide whether or not you should go surfing. The first step is to explore. When a person comes to see us for the first time, we need to initiate a connection. This is what I call *yogayoga*.

Unfortunately, we sometimes mistakenly assume things. I always say, when you meet someone, don't think you know everything. You have to follow the body and clear the mind, and sometimes you have to test the situation and the student, just as you'd test the soil. Where our test results are positive, the chances for change are good. In ancient times, the teacher would always test the student. He would check for things like honesty and sincerity. Sometimes the teacher would leave something around on purpose and then ask the student, "Did you find anything here?" If the student answered, "There was nothing here, sir," then the teacher would know that the student was a liar. On the other hand, if the student stayed on the spot to protect the property of the teacher, then the teacher would know this was an honest person. These tests were done to assess the quality and character of the student. Something of great value should not be given to a person who cannot appreciate it. Diamonds should be given only to someone who is responsible enough to have them. Do you also test patients in your work?

H: Psychoanalysts never manipulate a situation or a person in their work. But I use information that people give me about their behavior in indirect ways. For example, if patients don't respect my time and consistently come either very late or very early, I can see that they are not able to work within the set framework of our relationship. I will have to ask myself whether I can work with them within my own framework. Or if they arrive a bit early, I usually let them go into my office and I leave them alone for a short time. When I enter the room for our session, I can see how they behaved while they were alone. Most of them will sit and wait. Some of them go around and look at everything, and some will take books out of my shelf and look through them. This behavior gives me information about the level of respect for appropriate boundaries they have toward others. Sometimes I pay attention to the ability of a person to schedule sessions or to come to appointments at times that are not convenient for them. Also, when patients miss a session without prior cancellation, I ask them to pay for the missed appointment. It should be understandable that they pay in some way for the inconvenience they caused. I wouldn't force them to pay, but in the course of a discussion I would try to understand how they perceive the situation and try to understand it with them on this basis. The way people handle these kinds of issues tells me a lot about their capacity to take care of themselves as well as others. In the course of our sessions, a feeling of joint responsibility for our work and our time schedule should emerge. I consider these things as important indicators for the quality of our working relationship. I've found that people who are able to stick to certain inherent rules in relationships have a better chance of developing than people who are not able to do this. I consider it an important step forward when a patient becomes able to take responsibility for his or her commitments to me. But as I said, I won't manipulate a situation; a simulated or artificial test only makes a situation more complicated.

D: In the next sutra, Patañjali presents an analogy of how change occurs using the example of a farmer:

> *nimittam aprayojakaṁ prakṛtīnāṁ varaṇa-bhedas tu tataḥ kṣetrikavat*
> Such intelligence can only remove obstacles that obstruct certain changes. Its role is no more than that of a farmer who cuts a dam to allow water to flow into the field where it is needed. (YS IV.3)

Kṣetrika means "a farmer" or "a gardener." A farmer is not the seed, nor is a farmer the water, the soil, the sand, or the wind. But a farmer knows about these things. He knows the quality of the soil, he knows where water can be found, how to transport the water, he knows when he must give water and how much, he knows if the water is clean, he understands the properties of the soil, which types of seeds should be grown and when, what must be given to the soil, and in what way. A farmer pays constant attention to the soil, the water, the seeds; he is always watching. If there are weeds, they must be removed. If there are insects that are not good for the plants, he may have to use certain methods to remove the insects. So everything is present, but the farmer adjusts things so that the soil and the seed will produce the best fruits or flowers possible. The farmer is a catalyst. This is what we call *nimitta*. *Nimitta* is someone who knows, not someone who has. Creation consists of two parts. One part is the source—for example, the seed—and the other part is somebody who knows how to use it. Another example is a potter and the clay. Without the clay there can be no potter, and without a potter the clay cannot be transformed into anything. Without any wood, how could a carpenter make a table? And without a carpenter, how could the wood be used? Everything is already there, but somebody has to find out how to use what is there. This is what the third sutra says: Changes happen as in the presence of a farmer; everything is there, and the intelligence applied by the farmer enables the plants to grow. The farmer here is one who knows and one who acts. He is giving not just anything, but that which is needed. Everything is already there, but without his help there would be no plants.

H: What a beautiful picture! But I would like to ask something. *Nimitta* is described here as being active, as someone who knows. However, you used the image of a catalyst, which is itself something passive in that change happens solely due to the presence of the catalyst.

D: A catalyst is not a very good example. *Nimitta* is active; that is why the term *kṣetrika* is used, which means someone who works actively in the fields. *Kṣetra* means "field," and *ka* means "one who acts." So this is not a passive force, it signifies something active: the one who acts in the field.

H: So this means that the farmer takes care of his plants?

D: Yes, he is in a relationship, he is connected and takes care of what needs to be done. For example, in the kitchen there is rice, there are vegetables, there is everything, but there is no food until the cook enters and cooks. The cook is not the rice, not the vegetables; the cook is the one who knows: a dynamic, intelligent force.

H: But how does *nimitta* know, for example, the quality of the soil? He must have had his own experiences; he must have lived in the field?

D: Yes, exactly. This is why *kṣetrika* is also called an *ācārya*. *Ācārya* does not mean a scholar but someone who has worked in a certain field and who gained his own experience. A farmer is not a farmer just by birth; he has to get training and have his own experiences.

H: At the same time, there is a kind of reciprocity between a farmer and his plants. The farmer will live near his fields; he will be affected by the plants. If they do not grow, he may be disappointed or depressed. He is constantly in touch with the results of what he is doing, and this has an effect on him.

D: Yes, of course. The farmer is someone who is totally focused, just like a yogi. This Sanskrit word was also used in the Bhagavad Gītā to refer to a yogi.

H: At the same time, there is also the idea of devotion. The farmer is devoted to his fields and his plants.

D: Yes, exactly. I have met farmers who were that devoted. Sometimes they even pray to God to ask for rain so that the plants can have some water.

It is said if the farmer is good, the yield will be good. If the farmer is not good, even though there may be good manure, good seed, good water, and so forth, still the yield will not be good. In our interaction, it is almost the same. The teacher is like a farmer, and the student is like the field. Let's take another example. In Israel, nothing grew near the Dead Sea because there was too much salt in the soil. Some scientists did research and found out that when they removed the top layer of soil, the soil below was very good. Today, some of the best flowers and best vegetables are grown near the Dead Sea. The farmer in this case includes the scientists who helped it become a fertile place.

So we see that *nimitta* is like the teacher and the field is like the student.

H: This picture of a gardener or farmer indicates a relationship in which someone is constantly connected with his work. This is a living relationship.

D: Correct. That is why the word *kṣetrika* is used: someone who is in contact with the soil. It is not the word *kṣetrajña*, "one who knows." He is not an agricultural scientist, he is a farmer. There is a big difference between an agricultural scientist and a farmer. An agricultural scientist in Sanskrit is called *kṣetrajña*. This is someone who knows everything about the soil, but often only in a theoretical way. The agricultural scientist often doesn't even know how to dig the earth. But the person who really knows the soil is the farmer. The scientist has to communicate to the farmer. A *kṣetrajña* should aid the *kṣetrika*, who is the farmer. Often, a *kṣetrika* is a humble person, whereas a *kṣetrajña* is an arrogant person.

Let us move to the next sutra, which honors people who work with the mind:

> *nirmāṇa-cittāni asmitā-mātrāt*
> With exceptional mental faculties, an individual can influence the mental states of other beings. (YS IV.4)

Nirmāṇa means "reconstruction"; *citta* means "the mind." How can the mind be reconstructed? How does this work? The sutra discusses this phenomenon.

The word *asmitā* occurs here as well; interestingly, we find the term *asmitā* in every chapter of the Yogasūtra. In the first chapter, we find the term *asmitā* in sutra 17; in the second chapter, it is listed as one of the *kleśas*; in the third chapter, it is one of the *saṁyamas*; and in the fourth chapter, it is here. *Asmitā* is a Sanskrit word that comes from *as*, the verb "to be." *Asmitā* is the state where I am *with something*, linked to something.

This connection develops when we meditate. First we have a superficial connection. Then we get to something deeper and more subtle. When we enter into a profound connection, we discover something profound within ourselves: deep joy, also called *ānanda*. Ultimately, the connection may develop to the extent that I as the meditator and the object I am meditating on become one. It is almost as if we could not say which is this and which is that. The soil and the water are so mixed that we don't know which is the soil and which the water. This is *asmitā*.

H: This is some kind of fusion?

D: Yes, absolutely. To reconstruct the mind, there should be a strong link between the person seeking change and a leader or guide who can help direct that change. This sutra emphasizes a deeper relationship with someone who has higher inner resources and qualities. The Sanskrit word for "leader mind" is *nāyakacitta*. *Nāyaka* means something like "a leader." As a psychoanalyst, you are also a *nāyakacitta*. And the person who comes to you is looking for change. So *nāyakacitta* means "a mind at a higher level." It is not enough for me to come and sit in front of you even if you have a mind at a very subtle level. If there is no *asmitā*—or in other words, if there is no deeper connection—then there can be no transformation. There may even be this deeper connection to different people at the same time. When there is a strong connection, there may be a change in the mind *because* of this connection. Transformation happens differently to different people depending on their characters and inclinations. But there must be a leader who can provide the chance for transformation.

H: Would you say that this is because they identify with the character of the leader or teacher, and that they want to be one with that person or to become like that person?

I can give you an example of how we see such situations. A patient of mine caused me to worry and be fearful about his health for quite a long period of time. He constantly maneuvered himself into dangerous situations where his life was at risk. I became aware that he was observing my reactions to his experiences. I was in a difficult situation. Had I told him to stop putting himself into dangerous situations, he would have interpreted this as my fear. He could have interpreted such behavior as meaning I did not trust him to be careful and to take responsibility for his own life. However, had I not reacted at all, that might have come across as lack of interest. At an opportune moment, I commented that I felt he was observing me to see how I dealt with the situation. The patient took this as a chance, despite external pressures, to establish an inner freedom that enabled us both to reflect on what was happening to him. My attitude of inner freedom was something he could identify with, and this in turn gave him the inner freedom necessary to develop himself further.

D: Yes, this is also possible in yoga. For example, yesterday I saw a doctor who had back problems. He had been living in the United States and is having trouble adjusting to life in India again. He has a wife and two children and can't find a job here. I gave some instructions to his yoga teacher and asked the teacher to follow my suggestions. At the end of the lesson, the doctor's back problems had come back and were so bad that he could not get up. The teacher could not do anything, so he asked me for help. I went to the room and the doctor said to me, "I can't get up. I don't know what to do. Tomorrow we have a very important meeting. I don't know how I will get there." So I said, "In one minute you will be all right. I will do some chanting for you." So I took his hand and started chanting for him. I recited a text on the moon and planets. Then I said, "Now you can get up." I touched the part of the body where he had the pain. In five minutes, he was able to get up. He asked somebody to get him a taxi. One hour later, his wife called me to say he was well and to thank me. This was possible because he trusted me: I had seen him regularly for a number of years, so we had an old connection. This is *nirmāṇacitta*. He had so much confidence and faith in his *citta* that his mind was transformed from fear to faith within five minutes. That is *asmitā*, what you have called "identification."

H: When your hands touched him, that might have been symbolic of being in a very deep relationship with you. But why was he unable to stand up? Was it only fear?

D: It was also a physical problem. He had had this problem three years earlier. This time fear was also a factor. It is the same with children. When my granddaughter falls down, she cries and is afraid but doesn't want anybody besides me to pick her up. Transformation requires a connection to someone, a relationship with deep faith and confidence.

H: The idea of confidence and connection is far deeper than our concept of identification. For example, I can identify with someone without being touched by this person. Here, it seems that the inner connection plays a crucial role.

D: This is true.

H: Then the question arises as to how the teacher can approach someone in order to provide the possibility of a deep connection to aid transformation. This is a problem not only for the person involved, but also for the teacher.

D: Absolutely. There are three types of connection. One is the connection of the student with the teacher. Then there's the teacher's connection with the student. Finally, there is mutual connection, which is the ideal. The teacher moves toward the student, and the student moves toward the teacher. This is not a passive process.

H: The student and the teacher must suit each other. We call this "matching." Not every student matches every teacher.

D: Yes. The dynamic of this must come from both sides.

H: This sounds like our concept of effectiveness in psychoanalysis. There are psychoanalytic studies in which scientists have looked for criteria that would predict the results of psychotherapeutic treatment. Do you know what they found out? The single criterion that could predict a positive outcome of therapy was the level of matching between the patient and the therapist. In cases where there was a good level of matching—in other words, where the therapist and the patient were compatible—there were better results from the therapeutic treatment; this was independent of the level of severity of the illness.

D: Exactly.

H: The capacity of a teacher depends on his or her ability to make the relationship fit. The role of the student is to develop a sense of confidence and to be willing to grow in the process.

Can you say something more about *asmitā*?

D: *Asmitā* in this context means a heart-to-heart connection. This is very important. People often ask me, "What is *asmitā*?" I tell them that *asmitā* is a heart-to-heart connection; it is not merely an intellectual connection.

H: So *asmitā* seems to have a double meaning. On the one hand, it means the "I-ness," the uniqueness of what I am, and the merging with this "I" or with what I am. On the other hand, it describes an emotional relationship, as you have explained it here.

D: *Asmitā* has different meanings in the various chapters of the Yogasūtra.

In the first chapter, *asmitā* means I am meditating on something; slowly I become one with the object of my meditation. This is the highest state of yoga. Two become one.

In the second chapter, *asmitā* means there is an "I" and my habits or conditioning, also called *saṁskāras.* Here, the merging is between the "I" and my habits, because past conditioning and habits dominate. This means that the habits become the boss as I identify with my habits. The real "I-consciousness" is almost like a slave of this process. This is what we call *avidyā*.

In the fourth chapter, *asmitā* is again different. Here is a situation where there are lots of people and one master, and people are linked to the master so strongly that they almost cannot be separated. Here *asmitā* is something that contributes to change, helps transformation. So in the first chapter, it is an identification with an object; in the second chapter, the identification is with habits; and in the fourth chapter, the identification is with a leader or a teacher.

H: So at any rate, it seems that *asmitā* implies a certain merging with something.

D: Yes. The word *asmitā* comes from the words *aham tat asmi*, which means "I am that I have become one with."

H: It is like children who try to become like their parents through imitating the behavior of their parents.

D: Exactly.

H: This kind of identification is a critical part of a child's development. Whatever one does later in life, this tendency of a child to want to be like his or her parents will have an effect on the child.

D: In the first chapter, *asmitā* refers to something we freely choose. In the second chapter, it refers to our habits. Now here in the fourth chapter, *asmitā* refers to the relationship we have with someone whom we respect and trust.

In all of these cases, transformation is not meant to be merely intellectual, but involves every cell of the body. This sutra emphasizes that to achieve positive transformation, our effort alone is not enough; we need guidance. That is what you also do in Western psychology.

H: It is similar, but it seems yours implies something even more. In Western psychology, we try to be like partners on similar levels. What you are saying is that it is not possible to really help people in the process of transformation if one is on the same level they are. Something essential that can be aspired to should already be present in the teacher or in the psychotherapist—a kind of necessary asymmetry, if I understand you correctly. The student or the patient then develops a desire or even a hunger to become like the teacher, to aspire to develop the qualities perceived in the teacher or therapist. The teacher or therapist must already have these qualities the student or patient seeks to have.

In psychoanalysis, we speak about the phenomenon of "transference." This means that our patients project certain inner images onto us. We as therapists become an expression of their inner worlds, which they may love or hate. Sometimes we stand for the father, the mother, or a sibling, for example. Sometimes they imagine we are an ideal person into which they would like to transform themselves.

D: This special quality of the teacher is not something one can expect or want to have; we earn these qualities through love, respect, and sincere trust.

H: So a yoga teacher already should have developed certain qualities or perhaps have certain innate qualities or gifts. This would mean that one cannot become a yoga teacher through a training program?

D: I believe what you are saying to be the case. If I want to share honey with others, I must produce honey myself. Without producing honey, how can I give any away? And to produce honey, I must also apply effort. My father always said that we must deserve our position by our own efforts and example. We should not simply preach to others. We have to put in tremendous effort to deserve this role. That is what an *ācārya* is.

H: The most important point here seems to be the idea of authenticity on the part of the teacher.

D: Yes, exactly, that is a good word. Authenticity is essential. Shall we go on to the next sutra?

pravṛtti-bhede prayojakaṁ cittam ekam anekeṣām
This influence also depends on the state of the recipient. (YS IV.5)

There is one *citta* on one side and many different *cittas* on the other side. There is only one leader and many different minds centered on his or hers. These different minds are not identical; their mental situations are different. This is called *pravṛtti-bhedam*; *pravṛtti* is a movement, action, or activity.

My daughter and I once went to the cinema to see a Hindi film. Since I don't understand Hindi, I was mainly interested in the technology of the cinema, while she understood everything and was involved in the emotional story. So it was the same situation, but also different experiences at the same time. What she received was different from what I understood. I learned a lot about the technology producing the film. She was involved in the plot. The same environment, the same focus, the same connection, but each one in a different situation. What we received was therefore also different.

In a similar way, transformation happens to different people in different ways depending on individual connections, interests, tendencies, and states of mind. For example, when I look at our garden, I see the butterflies. My wife, on the other hand, looks to see if the plants have been properly watered. I am always fascinated by the butterflies: How do they come, and how do they know where to go? My attention is on the butterflies. My wife never even sees them. She is looking at something else. I am one mind, and she is a different mind. What she and I receive are different. Transformation is not identical; it is individualized.

H: In psychoanalysis, we call this "the inner world" in which a person lives. Everyone lives in his or her own inner world, which we at first have to understand. We need many sessions to begin to develop a common language with the patient. We know that each patient sees something different in us. For one person, we may represent the father figure who implies security; for the next, we might be a brother with whom the patient competed; for the third, we might be a sister who always took away his favorite possessions. We call this "projection" when the patient places inner pictures onto us. We become like a screen onto which the patient can place his or her inner images or desires. In psychoanalysis, we consider it a fascinating aspect of life that people see things in such different ways. A large part of our work consists in finding out how our patients perceive themselves and others and then discussing this with them.

I have a question: How do you see this individualized process of perception working within groups?

D: Even if there is a group, the process of change happens differently with different people. The next sutra says the following:

> *tatra dhyāna-jam anāśayam*
> Influence on another by one whose mind is in a state of *dhyānam* [meditation] can never increase anxiety or other obstacles. In fact, they are reduced. (YS IV.6)

What this means is that transformation per se need not always be identical for all people. What is good for some people may be dangerous for others. Transformation is not necessarily always growth. It could be anything: positive, negative, pleasant, unpleasant, constructive, destructive. However, this sutra clarifies that in a situation of *tatra dhyāna-jam anāśayam*, meaning when the person is linked to a positive force, then something positive will happen. That is why information can be given to one thousand people at the same time, but to establish a relationship, we must have a one-to-one connection and we must know the student.

For example, yesterday I met an Indian lady whom I had first known twenty-eight years ago. She lives in America now. She wanted to see me, so she came to India. When I saw her again, I could not recognize her. My memory, however, told me something like "I know her." She used to be lean, but today she has become overweight because of thyroid problems. So I paid attention, tried to concentrate, and said, "Hello, how are you?" She could hardly walk. It took me half an hour to establish a connection with her. For five minutes, I just closed my eyes and did some chanting for her. Then I opened my eyes. She was completely in tears. At this point, we were connected again. Only then did we begin to speak about her situation.

This is what the next sutra says: How can I help somebody to grow without a connection to the person? This is what is meant by the term *dhyānam*. I must meditate on the person; I must get connected to that person. This connection must be to the person today, in front of me, not to the person I remember. The past is not the present. Her name is the same, but her being may be very different. That is why my father said that yoga was like surgery. You cannot conduct surgery at the same time on several people. A surgeon can help only one person at a time.

This sutra tells us that the connection with the person must have total attention, *dhyānam*. If the student receives total attention, he or she will have less fear and insecurity. *Āśayam* means "I am in trouble, I could die . . ." This is *āśayam*: the feeling of, "I want to leave, I don't want to lose everything." *Anāśayam* means the opposite of this: "I am much better. Thanks to my connection with the teacher,

I am more confident. I am clearer and more at ease." For this to happen, there should be a connection. The teacher must be connected to the student, who must also be connected to the teacher. This is *dhyānam*.

In my own experience, it is not possible to be in a state of *dhyānam* if the mind is agitated. Even the teacher is no longer a guide in this situation. The student must be in a quiet state of mind. The teacher must also have a quiet mind and must understand the student as he or she is now. This is *dhyānam*, where you have a focus on something and where you are totally focused on that and nothing else. In this state, you can learn everything about the subject of focus. This is meditation.

We are also taught that this interaction between the teacher and the student is only for four ears. Two ears of the teacher and two ears of the student participate, and nobody else's. This individual relationship should be totally confidential. Nobody else should listen.

The first step in this process should not be taken by the teacher. The first step should be made by the person who is seeking help. The teacher should not go to someone and say, "I can help you." The person must say, "I would like to meet you, I would like to have a connection with you, may I please meet with you?" Then we can proceed. The initiative must come from the seeker. What is your view on this?

H: In psychoanalysis, it is the same. We also need the motivation and drive to come from the patient in order to begin. You are completely right: unless the first impulse is generated by the patient, we cannot start. The desire for change or the wish for help must be present. This is a requisite foundation on which to begin our work.

You also mentioned a further aspect that is important for psychoanalysis: we must have a structure for setting agreed-upon conditions for the duration of the treatment.

Initially, we try to understand why the patient has come to us. Once we have understood that, we can usually infer what he or she would like from the therapist. Still, it is important for us to articulate expectations and desires so that we can establish a reasonable working relationship. Once this is done, we agree to other details, including the costs of the treatment, the frequency of the sessions, and so on. We call all of these factors "the setting." Without an agreed-upon setting and without fixed rules, it is very difficult to establish and develop a stable relationship.

In addition to the patient's expectations and desires, which we have to discuss openly, the patient will often have related unconscious fears and anxieties that we can deal with only in the course of therapy as we become aware of them.

D: Yes, but sometimes we have to create confidence also. It is not enough to close the door and stay with the student. Some people are afraid of this kind of connection. We should be open and reduce their inhibition to ask questions.

H: Again I agree with you. A peaceful and calm environment is important so that the patient can feel at ease and find it possible to develop trust.

We try to talk with our patients early on about their fears. Sometimes this is not enough. Then we need to do something else. I would like to give you an example before we go on to the next sutra.

A female patient came to me because all of her previous relationships with men had ended badly. She wanted to have a family, but she had the impression that men generally treated her badly and then left her. The patient was attractive, intelligent, and successful in her job. So it was not easy to understand why she had continually had such bad experiences with the men in her life. It seemed apparent, however, that she had a deep-rooted problem in her emotional life that she was not able to solve simply with some easy words of advice. She had already tried all the tips and suggestions her friends had given her, to no avail. So I offered her a treatment of psychoanalytical psychotherapy with three sessions per week. She seemed desperate to find a solution to her problem. At the same time, she was afraid of getting dependent on me and of ending up disappointed in our work together if she engaged in a longer-term relationship with me. She hesitated and said that it would be too much of an effort for her to come and see me three times a week in addition to working at her job. I observed that she seemed to fear any kind of binding closer relationship and that this might be one of her problems. She then remembered a vacation she had had in Africa. She had wanted to experience the desert, but at the same time she had been afraid. In the end, a Berber suggested that he accompany her to show her part of the desert so that she didn't need to be afraid. I acted on this example and offered her a trial treatment of twenty-five sessions, after which she could decide whether she wished to continue with a longer course of psychoanalysis or not. She found this offer open enough and agreed. However, after twenty sessions had ended, she became nervous. She wanted to know if the offer was still good and if she could still continue with a longer course of treatment. Only once I had assured her that we could indeed continue and that my offer was still valid and that we could continue as we had done did she become calm again. She was silent for quite a while, and then she said that she felt calmer and more relaxed than she had in a very long time.

This shows that we need to react to our patients and their fears in an appropriate way. However, it also shows that that which patients fear can become valuable when they are able to overcome their fear. At the end of the trial sessions, my patient was afraid she would not be able to embark on longer-term psychotherapy treatment. She was then in a similar pattern from her past of fearing rejection.

Sometimes we need to perceive and understand certain fears in our patients at the outset of treatment and deal with these fears before we can establish a solid foundation.

If somebody knocks on the door, it is important that we answer in a friendly way. Sometimes, however, it is not enough to be friendly and open. We must then be able to share an experience with the patient in which the patient is able to show us his or her fears in a real and understandable way.

Now I think you wanted to speak about the topics of security and trust between a yoga teacher and his or her student as it is presented in the next sutra?

D: The next sutra reads as follows:

> *karmāśuklākṛṣṇaṁ yoginas tri-vidham itareṣām*
> And they act without any motivation, while others who also have exceptional capabilities act with some motivation or other. (YS IV.7)

The *yogī*, or the yoga teacher, is the person who helps us to transform. Patañjali uses the word *yogī* here. There are four types of yogis as described in this sutra:

1. *akṛṣṇa aśukla*
2. *kṛṣṇa*
3. *śukla*
4. *kṛṣṇa śukla*

The best yogis are *akṛṣṇa aśukla*. You can completely trust such a yogi. In Sanskrit, *kṛṣṇa* means "dark" and *śukla* means "bright." *Kṛṣṇa* refers to dark yogis; these are people who can harm you. They can cheat you or scare you; they create fear. There are examples where someone threatens someone else with black magic if that person doesn't do what is asked. *Śukla* yogis are people who do you good; however, they expect something from you. "I have done this for you, so now you must give me your house [or car or whatever]." People who are *kṛṣṇa śukla* are like those who are suffering from bipolar depression. Sometimes they act like a dark yogi, sometimes like a bright. The three last categories of yogi expect or demand something from you.

But yogis who are *akṛṣṇa aśukla* are neither dark nor bright. They offer something to others. They do not exploit anyone, and they do not expect anything. They are also called *sanyāsins*. Their actions are performed as a duty, without any expectation and without making a promise. They will never say, for example, "It is because of me that you got this."

H: They are neutral.

D: Yes, completely detached. They serve, but they would never say, "I did this for you." Their actions are for God or for freedom. *Karma* here means "action." They are active, and their actions are carried out in the sense of *Īśvara-praṇidhāna* with the idea that "it is our duty to do that." They don't play a game about being a "guru" or something. This is called *dharma yoga* in the Bhagavad Gītā: we have the right only to act, not to the fruits of our action. What will happen is not in our hands. This is a very high ideal indeed. If a student returns and says, "Thanks to you I can finally sleep well," this yogi would say, "It is not because of me. It is because of your efforts and your practice." Or the yogi might say, "It is a blessing from God, but it is not from me. You asked me to do something. I did that." Similarly, Jesus Christ said, "It is not because of me, it is because of your faith."

Kṛṣṇa yogis can be very dangerous. Sometimes they manipulate. And the others, *śukla* yogis, although they do some good, they can exploit people. For example, they might say, "I gave you so much, you must give so much; if you give little, I will only give a little." Patañjali presents four types of yogis here. Transformation, if it happens, depends not only on the student; it also depends on the quality of the teacher.

H: In this context, I would like to refer to the British psychoanalyst Wilfred Bion, who said that during the analytic session, the analyst should not have any personal desires or wishes: he or she should just be present and follow the words of the patient. What also seems important to me, however, is that the analyst or therapist does not allow him- or herself to be manipulated by the patient. The patient may praise the therapist or offer gifts. It is clear to us as psychoanalysts that the patient is under the influence of his or her relationship with us. We call this "transference," which means that the patient is not internally free or unbound. In this situation, if we accept a significant gift, we would be abusing the therapeutic role we have established. If the patient also thanks us profusely and says, for example, "Now I have a reason for living again, and I owe it all to you!" we can thank the patient for placing trust in us, but without identifying ourselves as being responsible for this change. We see the situation as an expression of the work we did, and we avoid the temptation of trapping ourselves within the transference established with the patient. We have to know how to deal with smaller gifts from a patient. Do we accept them or refuse them? If we accept them, we risk being manipulated; however, if we refuse even a small gift, we risk insulting the patient, making the patient feel rejected. A solution sometimes is to accept the gift so that the patient can express his or her thanks; then we put the gift aside and keep it for the patient. We can also try to interpret the meaning of the gift. Some patients try to test our ability to withstand their gifts. There are patients who try to tempt us with interesting offers or invitations. Again, we have to resist and to make our patients aware that we are not there to be entertained by them. Our goal in therapy is to enable patients to understand and help themselves, not the other way around. There are many ways of creating dependency and of bypassing the therapeutic situation. Sometimes it happens in a very subtle way.

D: I've had these experiences quite often. Here's an example. In 1967, J. Krishnamurti, whom I was teaching at the time, asked me, "Why do you have to teach all these people? You should be studying with your father." In fact, at this time I did really want to learn everything possible from my father. "I will pay you three times what you earn from teaching yoga every month if you focus only on studying with your father," he told me.

H: Did he make this offer while he was your yoga student?

D: Yes. He felt he had received so much good from it that he wanted to give something in return. I was earning six hundred rupees a month, and Krishnamurti said, "I will pay you two thousand rupees a month." Two thousand rupees in those times was a large amount; you could buy a scooter for that money! However, my conscience said, "No." I told Krishnamurti, "Thank you for your offer, but I don't want to accept your scholarship. I want to stand on my own two feet. I want to be independent." He asked why. "The moment I accept something from you, I will become your slave. And at the moment I become your slave, I will not have the authority to communicate with you." He was very touched.

Here is another example. At a moment when we had a serious political crisis in India, a European student of mine suggested I come to Europe. "You will have a nice apartment here. You will be able to live here with your family." This was very generous of him. He had an influential position, and he offered me many options to help me and my family. I refused. Imagine if I had accepted. I would have become a beggar. Even now, there are so many people who say, "What can I do for you?" I say, "Your best wishes are the best gift for me." The moment we accept such offers, our spiritual authority will be destroyed. We never know what will happen tomorrow. *Pariṇāma* (continual change) is always a factor.

H: In psychoanalysis, therapists see it as their role to be the guardian of the relationship. We must protect our working relationship so that it remains stable, appropriate, and vibrant. Only then can we be truly helpful to our patients. To ensure this, the International Psychoanalytical Association has set up guidelines to rule behavior with patients in therapy, and it expects all analysts to abide by these. The guidelines include passages that preclude therapists from accepting significant gifts, from embarking on business relationships, and from entering into sexual relationships with patients, for example. In individual cases, each therapist must decide for him- or herself how to apply these rules. Not an easy task!

D: In 1968, an American man came to study with me. He saw I had a scooter and he said, "You are my teacher; how can you drive on a scooter?" He went back to America and shipped a Volkswagen all the way to India for me. The car arrived, and the man said, "The car has arrived, so you must accept it." I said, "No. I will not accept it." In those days, to have a car like that was a very high status symbol. I said, "If I accepted the car, then every time I sit in it I will have to think of you. I don't want to think of you all the time. The only person I want to think of all the time is my teacher. So thank you for that, but I will not accept it." He was very sad. He had to sell the car in India.

H: Sometimes we even consider such tempting offers as a kind of aggression unconsciously directed toward the relationship. We have to resist this for the sake of the patient. The moment we accept, the whole relationship could be altered and possibly destroyed.

D: There is a beautiful expression: The hand that gives is always above the hand that takes. So the receiving hand is underneath. The moment I give something to you, you become like a slave. Professional relationships are different from sentimental relationships.

I want to be free. I don't want to be a slave. When I am a slave, I compromise.

H: But there is another problem. These people want to have the chance to express their gratitude. Perhaps they do this in one way by becoming healthier, but shouldn't there be another way for them to express their appreciation?

D: I always tell them, "The best gift you can give me is to continue to grow. That is the best gift. Because when I see you growing, it gives me so much joy. This gives me much more pleasure than a bank account ever could."

Now I have a question for you. Many people pose the following question: "How can I find the right teacher? The person whom I can trust?" Which also means as much as, how can they find the right teacher who will not manipulate and take advantage? "Can I assume that someone who is quite well-known is the right teacher?" This is a question I hear from many people coming from the West. How do you see this?

H: I would suggest that after they have met the teacher, people should look inward and try to find out how they felt when in contact with this teacher. Then they should reflect on how they felt the day after meeting the teacher. During their yoga studies or lessons, they should also reflect on how they are progressing or changing, take some time to observe. The most important question for me is whether there is some kind of development. And I would suggest trying to see if there is an inner space, a feeling for development and inner freedom, when they are in touch with the teacher.

D: My father composed a poem on this. In this poem, he first says that when we are agitated and mentally unquiet, that is not the time for a guide or teacher. First, quiet your mind. You might do this by some kind of relaxation or some chanting, for example. When the mind is jumping around, don't let it jump to your teacher. And then be clear about why you are looking for a teacher. Do you have any particular motivation or a goal? What is your goal? What are you looking for? Is it physical help, or peace of mind, or the growth of your spirituality that you seek to have? Be clear about this. And then when you are clear about this, go to a reference whom you trust and who knows the teacher, before you go to the teacher yourself. Don't go immediately to the teacher. Get some information from trusted sources who know the teacher. Only then should you make a decision to go to that teacher. And once you go to that teacher, do not immediately submit yourself to the teacher. Watch, test, and be attentive.

H: But in the end, how do you decide? Are there some criteria to help make this decision?

D: The teacher should not immediately start by instructing the student. The teacher must first get to know the student. The teacher must know what his or her strengths or weaknesses are. Only then should the teacher begin to give instructions.

Sometimes a person will ask me, "Can you teach me meditation?" "Surely!" I reply. Then I wait. I don't take any further step. The person may come back and say, "Sir, I just want to remind you." "Okay!" I answer. "Please come on Sunday morning at eight o'clock and we will take the first step." Then the person may say, "Oh, I have a breakfast meeting with my friends. Sorry, but I shall not be able to come." "Okay, enjoy your breakfast!" If the breakfast is more important than meditation, fine; however, somebody else may say, "Anytime you tell me to be here I will, because this is important to me."

A friend of mine wanted to learn meditation. After he made the decision to do this, I said, "Okay, please come on Friday at six o'clock in the evening. I'll teach you meditation." Later, his wife told me that he had been scheduled to give the keynote address at a conference in Bangkok. He canceled his participation because he didn't want to miss his lesson in meditation. He never told me about this; his wife did. I said, "Why didn't you tell me?" "That was of no importance, sir. This was more important." He still practices his meditation today.

H: He was obviously very serious and very motivated. But on what basis did he make this decision?

D: He had been looking for a teacher, and a friend of mine, whom I had known for fifteen years and who was also his friend, said to him,

"You can trust this man. He looks just like a normal person, but don't go by how he looks. He doesn't wear a long beard and he doesn't look like a Hindu. But go to him."

H: So it was due to his friend?

D: Yes, a very good friend. There were also some tests.

H: So in the end, what makes it possible to find the right teacher?

D: It is a bit like luck. I never imagined that I'd have such a deep and positive relationship with my father. I decided that I wanted to study with him. He was so patient with me. This was really my great luck. My elder brother also studied with my father, but he could not cope with my father and so he left home. My younger brother, who lives in France now, became my father's student even before I did. But somehow the connection was not very good. That is why he left India and went to France. I was a late starter, but my connection deepened and lasted nicely until he died. My mother never thought that I would be a student of my father's. My father and my mother were so proud that I was an engineer. In those days, that was something special in India. When I left engineering, my mother was worried about the loss of income. Yes, I must admit it was really a lot of luck for me. My father lived for more than one hundred years, and he taught me many things.

H: Even if it was luck, you must have also felt somehow that it was worthwhile to stay and to continue your studies. There must be something in the student that makes him or her stay?

D: I feel that at the same time we teachers must have a quality that instills confidence in the student. It is an effort we have to make. For example, when I asked my father how he could stop his heartbeat, he demonstrated it to me and thus proved it. This builds more and more confidence.

H: In the language of psychoanalysis, we would explain it like this: We strive to fit in to such an extent that the therapist can become a good object for the patient, as good as it was in the first days of the patient's life. We try to become a desired object, to fit into the pictures of the patient's inner world. We try to be useful and to be able to survive as a good object in our relationship with the patient.

D: Beautiful.

H: Yes, when it works, it really is a beautiful thing. But sometimes the patient cannot bear it, and he or she will try to attack this to repeat bad past experiences.

D: I often think about how some people who practice *āsana*, read the Yogasūtra, and work as yoga teachers or therapists still lead a sad life. I see something similar to what you are describing: some teachers or therapists are qualified, they might even do a lot of therapy on their own, but still their personal life is not happy. In these cases, the good object is missing.

H: If I understand you correctly, then the yogi must have access to his or her inner world to be able to find this positive object within him- or herself. The yogi should be linked to something that is entirely positive. Only then can the yogi establish and maintain a good relationship. The yogi is also then in a position to help others find this positive object within themselves someday.

D: This is what we call an *ācārya*. This kind of person is an example. *Ācāryas* have overcome problems themselves, so they know what they are talking about and how to solve problems.

Let us now look at the eighth sutra in the fourth chapter:

tatas tad-vipākānuguṇānām evābhivyaktir vāsanānām
Since the tendency of the mind to act on the basis of obstacles, such as misapprehension, has not been erased, these obstacles will surface in the future and produce unpleasant consequences. (YS IV.8)

I am sure as a psychoanalyst you will be interested in this. Let me start with an example, then I will come to the idea of the sutra.

There were once two friends who were very close. They were from different families, and they studied together at university. After that, both of them decided that they would go abroad, so they even went together. They went to the United States and first got their master's degrees, and then they were both hired to work in the same company. Let us call the one person Peter and the other person Paul. So Peter and Paul worked in the same company. They were both in the sales department. Paul had a knack for getting things done. He was able to speak to the clients very pleasantly; whenever he was involved in a sale, more goods were sold. Peter somehow was not a very good communicator. He was a bit shy, and sales in his section were not as successful. The boss was very impressed with Paul, whom he promoted. Within eight years, Paul had become the supervisor of his friend and colleague Peter. Peter became very jealous of Paul. He said to himself, "Somehow I must show the boss that Paul is not such a good fellow. Then I can get promoted and Paul will get demoted." In the company, there were ethical guidelines not to accept gifts from clients. So Peter found out the name of one of Paul's clients and sent Paul a gift addressed from this client. When Paul received this gift, he went to his boss and said to him, "Sir, what shall I do? We are not supposed to accept anything from our clients. I want to return the gift to him." So he phoned the client and he learned that this man hadn't sent him anything. Paul started to investigate where the gift might have come from. He went to the shop where it came from and found out that Peter had purchased it. He went to Peter and said, "I am so touched that you sent me this present. You didn't want me to know that it came from you. Now I want to give you something, too. Here is a brand-new car. You must accept it!" Peter felt so ashamed and began to cry. Then he confessed the whole thing and asked Paul to forgive him.

There is another story about Rāmānuja. When a great master of Vedānta found out that his student Rāmānuja had ideas that could endanger the whole system of Vedānta, he decided, together with his other students, to kill Rāmānuja. They led him to a dangerous place where tigers lived, and they left him there. But Rāmānuja was found by a hunter who saved him. Thus Rāmānuja was able to survive and develop his ideas.

This sutra says that deep inside us there are unexpected parts of ourselves that may come up in certain circumstances.

H: In psychoanalytic thinking, we have discovered that jealousy is one of the deepest motivations for destructive behavior. It is the most powerful complex in the human mind. It starts with Adam and Eve and their children Cain and Abel. When Cain realizes that the offerings of his brother Abel were accepted by God and that God obviously loved Abel, Cain becomes jealous of his brother and kills him. So in the Bible, the very first crime in human history was because of jealousy. We say it is the oldest and deepest source of destructiveness. In therapy, patients sometimes cannot tolerate the fruits of their work with the therapist and therefore feel the urge to destroy it by not progressing or by getting worse. We call this a "negative therapeutic reaction."

Another source of destructiveness is the fear that your own mental world, which you have constructed and established, will be destroyed. In other words, you can fear that the behavior or actions of someone else will destroy your own basic assumptions. This is apparent in the second story of Rāmānuja, who provoked deep fear with his new ideas, which threatened the whole system of Vedānta. The people in the story reacted out of a fear of being destroyed mentally by something they couldn't understand. The entire spiritual and mental existence of the teacher and the other students was at stake. In such situations, unexpected underlying destructive actions may suddenly surface. We must always be aware that something like this can happen. If I understand your examples correctly, this sutra speaks about very deep roots of fear and envy in us that can trigger unexpected and terrible behavior. Am I right?

D: Exactly. Some consequences of our actions relate to our previous habits and behaviors. When such things appear, it happens so fast.

H: This is rooted very deeply within us. These types of reactions happen very fast and are almost always unconscious.

We see in our work with patients an unconscious pattern of reacting that is rooted in their past history. Patients say that they often become involved in situations that anger them or in conflicts that escalate as the result of some unknown misunderstanding—no one knows why it happened. If we look closely at the situation, we can often see that the patient felt wounded or hurt in some way and reacted immediately without reflecting or even becoming aware of the situation. Often both the cause and the reaction are linked to a perceived insult from another person; however, generally the person is unaware of this. These kinds of reactions are rooted in us and very hard to change because they occur so quickly. Do you think that such behavior can be changed? How do you see this in yoga?

D: Yes; this is discussed in sutra 11. Change is not impossible. As you correctly say, however, and as the next sutra will show us, fear is a very strong factor here. Fear triggers certain behaviors. As an analyst, you know how powerful the ego is. The ego decides many issues.

H: In my opinion, we are talking about habits and reactions against which words alone are relatively powerless. These reactions come with such overwhelming force or speed that the so-called ego is helpless to do anything against them. I think certain qualities of the ego can be cultivated; there is no doubt about this. We psychoanalysts say that ego is a structure that aims to protect us against those older fears and impulses. The ego is a kind of reaction and defense against tendencies to destroy and to react. It is therefore a kind of cultivated response against uncontrolled impulses. What you are talking about here takes place in the foreground of such complexes within us related to envy, greed, and psychic wounds. Behind all of this is the deepest of all fears, the fear of destruction, which can no longer be cultivated. So this deals with unconscious reactions to the fear of destruction, which played a role even before our ego was fully developed.

D: That is why I never forget what Krishnamurti once told me: "Don't become another monkey. Be patient. Things will change." It is very easy to just become another monkey. We might think, "He is nasty, so I am becoming nasty. He is upset, he hates me, so how can I be nice to him? He cheated me, how can I not cheat him?" In 1967, Krishnamurti said to me, "What is the difference between you and the other person? Be patient. Things will change." I have never forgotten this. Many people I have dealt with have provoked me. I am patient, and I have faith. So many things have happened because of this.

H: Are you hinting that the only way to overcome these kinds of negative reactions is to have faith?

D: Yes, I think so.

H: In psychoanalytic theory, we assume that in the first three years of their lives, people acquire a foundation for their subsequent development that is linked to their experiences of trust and confidence. We refer to this as developing a basic sense of trust or self-confidence. This inner confidence or sense of stability depends on the level and quality of the relationship people had with their mother or with whoever was their primary caregiver, and to what extent they can actively access positive inner pictures as a result of this experience. If these early experiences were good and helpful and have been stably anchored, then people are able to develop a solid sense of security; they have the impression that there is something that protects and carries them. We call this a "positive internal object" and it is a result of this early relationship with one's mother or primary caregiver. Someone who has established a positive internal object within him- or herself will be more confident and will be less easily upset than someone who is less secure and whose experiences are less consistently positive.

D: The ninth sutra in the fourth chapter says the following:

> *jāti-deśa-kāla-vyavahitānām apy ānantaryaṁ smṛti-saṁskārayor eka-rūpatvāt*
> Memory and latent impressions are strongly linked. This link remains even if there is an interval of time, place, or context between similar actions. (YS IV.9)

For example, sometimes people say, "I will forget what happened at home, because I am in my office and I have to design something and I am so absorbed in that, I don't remember what happened in the house." Another example: I was in the United States teaching at a college I was visiting. One day I was supposed to give a lecture, and I had a very strong toothache. Before giving the lecture, I had excruciating pain. I went ahead and gave the lecture for one and a half hours, and during this time I never had any idea of my toothache. I had no tooth pains at all. Why? Because I was interacting with a lot of people. Then after I finished the lecture I got into the car, and suddenly the toothache was back. Once again it was so painful! In the course of our lives, we have to fulfill different roles. Each time we are different. We play these roles like actors on a stage. This is what is called *jāti*.

Deśa is this: When I am in India, we have a certain climate and a certain culture, so we slowly adapt to the culture and the climate. For example, we are used to eating with our fingers and sitting on the floor. Then we go to another country and another climate. We must adapt. When I am in Sweden, I wear jackets and socks and shoes. When eating, everyone uses knives and forks. This is what is called *deśa*. We must act according to the location or *deśa* that we are in. However, when we are in accordance with the *deśa*, this does not mean that everything else is forgotten.

Kāla means "time." Time here is not only physical time, it is also psychological time. When we are depressed, we are thinking about something sad, but when we become active, we forget about that. So the sutra is saying that there may be a change in our role, we may be in a different country, we may be in a different time, but although certain things appear to be lost to us, they are in fact never truly lost. The moment there is a memory, this memory gets connected to our habits, and we come back to the habits consistent with *jāti*, *deśa*, and *kāla*.

I recently had a meeting with some colleagues in the United States. As I was coming out of the meeting, I saw a young Indian woman whose mother I have known for twenty-eight years. Although this girl was born in America, as soon as I saw her Indian face, I spoke to her in Tamil. Obviously she couldn't respond. I immediately switched to English, and then we started a good conversation. As soon as I realized that this girl was not an Indian and was in born in America, I asked: "So, do you like John Kerry? Do you think that Kerry is going to be elected, or will it be Bush?" She knew more about Kerry and Bush than a person from India would. Because I could speak to her in her language and within her culture, we established a good connection. We became friends.

The sutra says here: That which appears is only the surface. It does not mean other things do not exist. Multiple things can exist in parallel. Things that appear to us are there according to this particular situation. Remember the example of Rāmānuja and his teacher. Even though the teacher loved his student, as soon as he realized that this boy could be a danger to him and his followers, he said: "I must destroy him." And he tried to kill him. So nothing is lost. Certain things may not be apparent, but depending on the situation, different memories may arise. According to the memories, similar *saṁskāras*, or habits, may take over. We function according to these *saṁskāras*.

H: How should I understand the term *jāti* here?

D: If I meet different people, I behave in different ways. At eight o'clock this morning I met a journalist, and I spoke to him in one way. Now I am with you, and I am speaking in a different way. At nine o'clock I had a meeting with other people, and I was different again.

H: So it sounds like a kind of role I have to play, depending on the situation and the environment?

D: Exactly.

H: Depending on the situation and the role I have to play, I will be different. Other things are not forgotten, but they move to the background. They will come back as soon as the appropriate situation arises. So my behavior and my memory are related to the situation I am in?

D: Yes. As my father used to say: We are like stage actors. One day I may be a villain, the next I may be a hero. In other roles I may be a comedian. It is almost like a computer: you visit this website, you get this information; you visit the other one, you get the other information. It is all available, but what will appear depends on which buttons I press.

H: And is it similar with *deśa*?

D: Yes.

H: And *kāla*?

D: Yes, *kāla* means "time" and also the memory of time. For example, when we get up in the morning, we might be in a certain mood. In the evening when we are tired, we will be in a different mood. In the morning we have a lot of energy, in the evening we are tired. Time and change are linked. It is not only the present time, it is a time period—for example, when we were young, when we are old; this is also *kāla*.

H: In these examples, time can be preserved or extended?

D: Yes. Just because there have been changes in our circumstances does not mean that the things that happened in the past are lost. There is really no gap at all. Similar circumstances will invoke similar memories, and similar memories will invoke similar *saṁskāras*. This is why one of the definitions of memory is "knowledge based on *saṁskāras*" (habits).

H: This way of thinking strikes me as very modern. Recently, neuroscientists have begun to study and discuss similar phenomena of memory. They have developed a concept of memory based on modern scientific discoveries. Memory was previously understood as a kind of container where the data went in and we had only to retrieve it again. But newer research in neuroscience shows that memory is highly dependent on context. Memory can no longer be understood as something fixed and stable. It is constantly building categories and shifting memory into new categories according to the situation we are in. We open up these categories according to each situation as it arises. Emotions are also linked to those situations; this means our emotions are part of the whole picture. So we can no longer say that memory is stored information based on knowledge. It is based on a whole situation, including emotions. Accordingly, experiences are stored away in a kind of filing system that depends on a particular situation. This seems very similar to what you have just explained.

D: As the sutra says, memory is based on experience, not on facts. The way I experience something may be very different from how you experience it. This is why everything is based on experience. And how we experience is based on our conditioning. You know, it is amazing to realize that the way we look at something is grounded in our habits. Many years ago, there was a nuclear scientist who would come to study with me. He would normally sit outside on the street for fifteen minutes before our lessons. I asked him why he waited outside. He replied, "I like to watch the construction. Here in India people use such simple things to cut stone and build things. This is stunning for me. I never get to see this." This man was interested in engineering, so he always saw things in the context of engineering because of his interests and habits. So you see, often our experience is shaped by our own *saṁskāras*.

H: According to this assumption, that memory is constantly changing depending upon our current experience, we would find different categories for things we have experienced before. This means that memory constantly changes due to new categories. Is this how you see it?

D: Yes, of course. Memory will change provided we have a fresh look at things. If we do not look at things openly, if we do not really listen, but instead assume that we already know things, then it will not change. That is what is meant when we say, Take a second look at something. If we look again even more closely, we have a chance of seeing what is, and when we see what is, then we will correct our memory. This is what is meant by sutra 43 in the first chapter.

The message here is, "Don't look only from one angle. Go around and see it from different perspectives; then you can know the truth." Sometimes, even when we are attentive, our understanding is distorted because of ideas we have about something (as per YS I.42). Even when we are in a state of attention, our initial perception can be distorted by inputs coming from our memory, imagination, and so forth, but we think what we are seeing is the truth. That is why the next sutra says: "Verify!" Verify by checking and by going around from different vantage points, again and again. Then memory can be corrected so that a process of growth takes place within memory. So memory in the beginning is based on distortions and mistakes. We must apply effort with a clear mind and not assume that we know everything already; that is important, never assume that you know. Start afresh, as if you didn't know. This can allow a change in understanding, so memory can then become corrected.

H: This sounds very scientific.

D: It is based on experience.

You see, when people are happy and everything is going well, they don't remember much. But when things don't happen in the way people expect them to, you know what happens: the past takes over. Then there are so many complaints!

From where do we get this tendency to perceive things in a certain way or to behave in a particular way? What feeds this conditioning in us? The tenth sutra gives an indication:

> *tāsām anāditvam cāśiṣo nityatvāt*
> There is a strong desire for immortality in all human beings at all times. Thus, these impressions cannot be ascribed to any particular time. (YS IV.10)

Many of these *saṁskāras* (behavioral patterns due to habits) and *vāsanās* (deep and unconscious tendencies and impulses) have no beginning. *Anādi* means "We don't know how it all started." We don't know why every human being, in fact every living being, is constantly wishing to continue to survive. *Āśiṣa* means "I don't want to die. I want to survive. I don't want to lose everything." The wish for survival is eternal. Because every living being has this wish for eternal survival, there is always a struggle, an attempt to hold on to things. This is the reason that many of our *saṁskāras* are maintained. This is also why there is constant stress, the so-called fight or flight response. As long as we have a strong attachment to our survival, we will be dominated by old *saṁskāras*. We cannot get rid of them. They will always be there. What do you think?

H: This seems to me to be a very deep truth. I think it is even true when it comes to the survival of ideas or philosophical concepts. People even try to make their ideas eternal. You told the story of Rāmānuja's teacher, who felt he had to defend his ideas and his philosophy to such an extent that he attempted to murder his own student.

In psychoanalysis, the theory of narcissism deals with the problem of survival. Narcissism is a way in which a person seeks to stabilize him- or herself. There are examples in which a person places his or her sense of self above all other factors by trying to get other people to express their constant admiration and praise. A further aspect of narcissism is that it acts as a defense against the fear of death. A person who develops narcissistic traits does everything possible to resist and protect him- or herself from aging, from change, or from anything else that threatens his or her sense of self. A famous character in literature aptly portrays this tendency: Oscar Wilde's Dorian Gray. Dorian Gray, a beautiful young English gentleman, makes the wish that he remain young and beautiful forever and that a painting of him age in his place. The painting, hidden away in an upstairs attic, ages instead. The novel vividly depicts the terrible fears of aging and death in a person suffering from narcissism.

The problem a narcissist has is that he or she is unable to love anyone else. Every act serves a desperate need for self-preservation. Such a person seeks to avoid expressions of love or devotion toward others, because this love or devotion would threaten that person's own self-centered system. To experience love, the narcissist must entice others to love him or her. The narcissist seeks to live forever and to control anything that deviates from his or her own plans and ideas.

D: A well-known yoga teacher had invited me to present something about *prāṇāyāma* and *āsana* in Switzerland. I spoke about breathing and explained, for example, that when we inhale, the movement starts from above and goes downward, and that when we exhale, we contract the stomach. As soon as I started to present this, to about two dozen important teachers, I noticed a number of them started to get nervous. They had never been taught about breathing and *āsanas* together. Also, they had always spoken about breathing practices using the example of pouring water into a bucket. When you pour water, you start to fill at the bottom, so they said that when practicing *prāṇāyāma*, you must start in the stomach and then move upward. Some people wrote vehement articles against my presentation. So you see again what happens: people are concerned with their survival. Similar things happen in science. When someone discovers something new, other scientists will not accept it because they fear they will lose their own ideas. This is what is meant by *āśiṣa*: "I don't want to die; I don't want to lose my position; I don't want to lose my ideas; I want to prevail." There are many examples, even in philosophy.

H: Yes, we have many artists and writers who have written about this phenomenon. One of them is, as already mentioned, Oscar Wilde. History also provides us with many examples. Galileo Galilei was forced by the church to recant his discoveries. Galileo wanted to prove that the earth was not the center of the universe, that instead the center was the sun. This discovery was not in line with the beliefs of the Catholic Church, which felt threatened in its role as the single authority on the truth. Galileo was forced to recant.

This fear of being threatened by someone else's achievements can be seen among powerful politicians and fanatical philosophers. We even see examples of this among some artists. Some people feel genuinely threatened when they encounter someone who demonstrates better skills or abilities than they may have.

So you see, this is a phenomenon that we can find in all areas of life and society. It involves extreme situations. The people involved feel it is a matter of life and death.

D: In 1960, when I presented the idea of drawing *āsanas* with stick figures, many people criticized my approach. Now everybody is doing it. A Canadian friend of mine, Michael Smith, and I made a book of illustrations of *āsanas* and *prāṇāyāma* using these figures. When we gave this book to a Hindu newspaper for a review, the journalists on the newspaper wrote: "This is not a book on yoga; it is a book on drawing. It should not be read by anybody. Yoga is not merely drawing, yoga is something more." You see, this again was *āśiṣa*. When somebody is more successful, it provokes mostly fear. We find this in philosophy, in painting, everywhere. Jealousy and fear are inherent qualities.

H: Yes, the fears of destruction and loss are great motivators in people.

D: There are exceptions, but the majority are like that.

H: The foundation of this behavior is a fear of change.

D: Yes, you are right. The next sutra is very interesting. We may ask whether there is any hope to reduce all this. Is there any at all? The answer is, yes! There is hope that we can reduce and, in fact, change this. Let's look at the next sutra:

> *hetu-phalāśrayālambanaiḥ saṅgṛhītatvād eṣām abhāve tad-abhāvaḥ*
>
> These tendencies are both maintained and sustained by misapprehensions, external stimuli, attachment to the fruits of actions, and the quality of mind that promotes hyperactivity. Reduction of these automatically makes the undesirable impressions ineffective. (YS IV.11)

Here, Patañjali explains the four factors that lead to the continuation of *saṁskāras*. He describes this situation as a table with four legs:

1. *hetu*
2. *phala*
3. *āśraya*
4. *ālambana*

The tabletop is the *saṁskāras* that are supported or nourished by these four forces. Let me describe these forces:

Hetu means "the cause." Suppose somebody had a bad experience that he or she can never forget. This person remains under the influence of this strong impression. The son of a friend of mine, for example, is terrified of cockroaches, and he is a doctor. When he was young, an older boy put a cockroach on his ear. It crawled into his ear and he got frightened; his mother managed to remove it. Today, this man is an eminent surgeon; however, he is still scared of these insects. The moment somebody even speaks about a cockroach, he gets scared. This is what we call *hetu*: certain experiences we had when we were young that have had a profound effect on us. These influences, and later experiences of stress, lead us to create certain habits, which in turn serve to further maintain the habits. There are many examples of this. You as an analyst know this well. These can also be good things that determine our behavior. The influences can be good or bad. Either way, previous profound experience determines our later behavior.

Then we have what is called *phala*: I do something and get some benefit or result from that. If that result is disappointing, it will reinforce my old *saṁskāras*, my habits. We will think, for example, "Again this is happening and again I am a failure! I put so much effort into this and still it is not working!" Whenever the results of our actions are not as we wanted them to be, or when things happened that we did not want, we experience this as counterproductive to our wishes. We become disappointed, and this nourishes our *saṁskāras*. So we call *phala* the "fruits" of our actions; they are the results of our efforts.

Āśraya is an interesting word. It means "something that supports me and helps me to act." What helps me to act is "mine"; the fruit of my actions is also "mine." We look at things differently depending upon the structure and the quality of the mind. Sometimes our mind is very calm and we look at things calmly. If the mind is agitated, we can quickly get upset. This is like a kind of mood that we can fall into and that can color everything we experience. People who are depressed tend to see everything in a depressed mood.

The last word here is *ālambana*. This means "support." When I practice yoga, I become calm and clear afterward. If I read the newspaper and find out that our cricket team has lost, I get upset. Things we are exposed to connect us to our *saṁskāras*, our old patterns or habits. This is what is called *ālambana*. For example, when we look at somebody we like, or when we look at certain flowers we like, old emotions or feelings can surface. Suppose you are walking on the street and you meet somebody who had cheated you a long time ago; the memory will immediately come back. When a memory suddenly comes back, we associate certain people with certain things. When I see you, I think of Germany or of Santa Fe or of Sainte-Baume, places we have previously met. Memory is linked by these kinds of processes, to our *saṁskāras*. And then the *saṁskāras* take over. This is what is meant by the term *ālambana*.

H: So this is something that comes from the outside and sparks something inside us. An example might be, for instance, a situation where a person comes to India for the first time and feels confronted with a situation he or she experiences as chaotic. This may trigger some of the person's own problems that are linked with internal chaotic situations, and which then awaken internal *saṁskāras* or patterns that are related to that.

D: This is what the sutra says: *Saṁskāra* is supported and maintained by these four forces. So how can we reduce *saṁskāra*?

Hetu cannot be reduced or changed. It is in the past, and we cannot change the past.

Phala may be changed by certain attitudes, for example by feeling *Īśvara-praṇidhāna*. This advises us not to expect too much. The more you expect, the more you may be disappointed. At times it is better not to expect anything than to have high expectations.

Ālambana advises us to be in good company, to avoid a negative environment. Good association is important.

Āśraya requires practice. For example, we can affect our mood through our own yoga practice using methods such as meditation, *prāṇāyāma*, chanting, and other means. *Āśraya* refers to our mood or attitude.

So although we cannot change *hetu*, we can build up a different culture or attitude so that the older ones become less effective. In the first chapter, sutra 50 says: "If a new *saṁskāra* becomes stronger, the old *saṁskāra* becomes weaker."

H: This is a broad concept—we can act at multiple levels at the same time. But where is the concept of *nimitta*, the person who knows us, here? During this kind of work, surely there should be someone we can refer to?

D: That is the million-dollar question. Ideally, I agree with you, and if we have a good friend or a guide or a person who knows a great deal, it can really help a lot. But in reality, such a situation requires a great deal of luck. Sometimes we are lucky enough to find such people. Other times people may have a good teacher, but they are not able to build up a good connection. That is why I said that we have to put in some effort. Definitely without *nimitta* it is not easy to identify and use our potential. To use our potential, somebody has to tell you that you have this possibility.

My father always said, "For *nimitta* to function, one must first suffer. Without suffering, a person will not look for a solution. Even if the best God is next to them, they will not ask for help." The Bhagavad Gītā shows us this. Initially, Arjuna had God right next to him, but he never learned anything from Krishna until he started suffering. He suffered and suffered. Finally, helpless, Arjuna turned and asked Krishna for help.

My father was very emphatic about this. He said that without suffering, nobody will look for a solution . . . *bhoga duḥkha*.

H: In a different cultural setting but at roughly the same time, Sigmund Freud said a similar thing about suffering and healing. He said we should be very careful about removing suffering too early. Psychoanalytic treatment is supported and encouraged by suffering. The goal of the psychoanalytic treatment is to become "able to love and work." This implies that suffering will ultimately be reduced to a normal level.

So in the end, we have a realistic outlook with a tangible result: development and transformation are indeed possible. Both yoga and psychoanalysis clearly show us this. So we can be optimistic, but we must also realize that this cannot happen without effort on our part.

For most people, development and transformation require ongoing effort. Unfortunately, most people are willing to do this only when their distress is so great that it has become unbearable.

It can be very helpful if we are able to find someone who can guide us by showing us the ways we can develop further. A relationship with someone who knows us and whom we trust can be significant in this process. The deeper and more meaningful this relationship is, the greater the impact it can have on our process of transformation.

D: Absolutely.

H: Now we are able to understand how and why transformation is possible. We can also see to what extent a stable and competent relationship can help a person to change, and how sometimes it is even essential.

Afterword

BY HELLFRIED KRUSCHE

We have oriented our remarks in this dialogue toward the classical texts on yoga and psychoanalysis. The main guideline for our discussion has been the interpretation of the Yogasūtra as presented by the great teacher T.K.V. Desikachar, which he first learned from his teacher and father, the legendary T. Krishnamacharya. Both of these names stand for authentic expertise in this yoga tradition. In a series of open and spontaneous discussions, we compared their traditional, classical commentaries with examples and applications from the world of psychoanalytical psychotherapy. These discussions make clear that yoga is a path to inner freedom. This path involves the practice of physical and mental techniques to cultivate discipline intended to allow the practitioner to avoid succumbing to external stimuli and to focus instead on his or her inner world. This process of turning away from the sense-driven external world involves the practice of concentration on a chosen object that becomes the focus of attention. This is the process of meditation. The result of this process is the discovery of one's own consciousness and the experience of inner freedom. Consciousness here is described as having qualities we could associate with light and vastness. At the same time, this consciousness has a dimension that transcends individual borders and is therefore connected with the world. Identifying with this consciousness allows the yogi or yogini to experience a state free of the impulses of habitual action. Someone in this state can freely decide both whether and how he or she will act. In yoga, this state is called *kaivalya*.

Psychoanalysis does not have a goal similar to this profound personal transformation aimed at attaining a kind of complete inner freedom from all restraints. Instead, psychoanalysis seeks to lessen suffering and to help make life feel more worth living. The goal of psychoanalytic treatment is to remove symptoms and illnesses caused by psychological factors.

Psychoanalysis uses methods that are, however, in many ways similar to those used by yoga. Both psychoanalysis and yoga are concerned with the development of an inner world. It has been proven that psychoanalysis succeeds when it can enable patients to open up an inner world where they enter into a relationship with their inner images. This inner world may help patients develop a kind of inner space where they can better understand themselves and their situation. This understanding is linked to language, and the words of this language are the vehicles for expressing their understanding. Verbal exchange about a patient's experiences and the ability to reflect on them are the means of extending awareness. It is also the way in which a patient shares these experiences with his or her analyst. Later on, a patient learns to perform this reflection independently and to enter into this kind of dialogue alone. The process of speaking and reflecting about him- or herself is the means of extending awareness, also called "consciousness" here.

There are some startling similarities between the fields of psychoanalysis and yoga. Both schools are based on methodical systems of knowledge. Both also speak about unconscious motives and impulses that influence human behavior and from which we can free ourselves only by applying various techniques and a system of discipline. Impulses are not seen as chaotic. They can be clearly defined. For example, the fear of death, greed, desire, and disgust are basic factors leading to unconscious actions. The human tendency to identify with aspects of the external world, and to try to hold on to these identities or connections, leads us to lose our connection to our own inner world. Subsequently, this deciding moment of identification is in both schools the factor that causes us to lose our inner freedom and hence the ability to develop further.

Both yoga and psychoanalysis see this loss of inner freedom as being accompanied by a state of mind in which the person can no longer clearly differentiate between the world of desires and the external world of temptations and promises. Reality is therefore perceived in a distorted fashion owing to one's own ideals and wishes. These entanglements are seen by both yoga and psychoanalysis as factors that hinder development and growth. If these problems are addressed in a consistent process over a period of time, change and growth may take place.

The most important similarity between psychoanalysis and yoga is the fact that growth seems to require a relationship with a significant guiding person. Both of these cultural systems assume that change requires time and effort. Only when the combined factors of a guiding relationship, time, and effort are present can true change take place.

The importance of this long-term relationship is an ingrained aspect within the yoga tradition as well as within psychoanalysis. Recent scientific research supports this link. Studies examining the efficiency of psychoanalytic treatment (catamnestic studies) have shown that the length and intensity of the patient-therapist relationship during treatment have directly influenced and thus had a significant impact on the intensity and the stability of change in the patient.

Our dialogue indicates that targeted inner change and development, or transformation, is indeed possible. For this to happen we need enough time, we need a solid, high-quality relationship, and we need to apply inner effort. This is true for all cultures, in the East as well as in the West.

It seems fair to assume that the areas where ideas and techniques from both yoga and psychoanalysis intersect deal with knowledge that transcends the boundaries of culture and time; in other words, these insights are timeless and transcultural.

Our dialogue has also revealed some dissimilarities. Yoga assumes there is a level of consciousness that transcends individual experience and that can be seen to have some kind of regulatory aspect. This consciousness is supraindividual and is also contained within all people. It has a timeless quality. It was always present and also has a dimension similar to light. It is the center of perception and can also perceive itself.

Psychoanalysis sees consciousness more simply as a function that is oriented toward language. It is described as the cone of light emerging from a lamp. It is not seen as something having any level of existence on its own. According to Freudian psychoanalysis, consciousness or preconsciousness is that which can or could be expressed in words.

There is a distinct and systematic knowledge of the effect and meaning of consciousness within psychoanalysis, such as the discovery of a system of unconscious motives and impulses. The effectiveness of this understanding in treating psychological illnesses as well as in interpreting and understanding the world of dreams and the world of literature has been widely proven. The knowledge of these forces has been shown to be useful and effective in helping patients develop more understanding.

In particular, psychoanalysis has developed a keen understanding about the unconscious dynamics within human relationships. Here, for example, there is a great deal of understanding about the extent to which transference and projection can play a role within relationships and how this can be worked on in a targeted and controlled way within a therapeutic setting. An area of key importance is the understanding of transference and the so-called countertransference as well as the handling of the appropriate setting.

Traditional yoga is anchored within a traditional hierarchical structure. There are strict guidelines regarding the transmission of knowledge. A relationship to a teacher who is him- or herself connected to a living tradition serves as a guarantee for the validity of what is taught. The effectiveness of yoga is therefore largely dependent on the quality of the relationship the student has with his or her teacher. The student is expected to be able to trust his or her teacher and to apply him- or herself to the learned techniques. This student-teacher relationship must be free from doubt, aggression, and negative attitudes of any kind. Trust is the foundation for development.

Psychoanalysis has a tradition of critical research and the controlled spreading of knowledge through institutions and societies that publish their findings to the wider scientific community, hence allowing open discussions to take place in public.

The doubt that a patient has toward his or her therapist and working through the ambivalence and negative attitudes toward the therapist are important parts of psychoanalytic treatment. Dealing with inner conflicts and aggressive impulses in the context of treatment is a basic principle within psychoanalysis. Trust is therefore more a result of treatment than a prerequisite.

It is fascinating to see how two systems that both seek personal transformation but could hardly be more different in terms of culture and time period nonetheless have similar perspectives and recommended actions regarding essential aspects of the nature of human development. However, as we discovered during the course of our discussions, there are also fundamental differences.

Much indicates that these two systems can complement and support each other. We both maintain that students of yoga can profit from psychoanalysis, and patients in psychoanalytic treatment can also profit from yoga.

We live in an age where a lack of time, human resource management, and cost reduction all continue to take on ever greater roles. There are even attempts to standardize processes of personal transformation.

In the world of modern medicine, technical equipment now stands in the center of treatment. Doctors must analyze numerous computer-generated sheets of facts on a patient, but they barely have time to get to know the actual person they must treat. In psychoanalysis, there are also demands for efficiency. This means that therapeutic techniques that reduce treatment time are preferred over more time-consuming methods. In the course of technological development and greater use of information technology in general, we have forgotten that the concrete human relationship remains an essential factor in the development and transformation of a person. In a constantly changing world, health cannot be maintained without the ability to develop and sustain a sense of inner and outer equilibrium.

In times such as these, it makes sense to look back to the oldest knowledge in our cultural history and see what kind of new orientation this might bring.

Yoga and psychoanalysis both indicate that we have the potential for inner transformation.

Both systems provide techniques and aids to support the development of inner balance. However, these techniques can be effective only if applied on an individual basis appropriate for a person in his or her particular concrete situation and within the context of a solid relationship.

BIBLIOGRAPHY

Antonovsky, Aaron. *Unraveling the Mystery of Health: How People Manage Stress and Stay Well.* San Francisco: Jossey-Bass, 1987.

Bion, Wilfred R. *Attention and Interpretation: A Scientific Approach to Insight in Psycho-Analysis and Groups.* London: Tavistock Publications, 1970.

Bowlby, John. *Attachment and Loss.* 3 vols. New York: Basic Books, 1969–1980.

Coster, Geraldine. *Yoga and Western Psychology: A Comparison.* Delhi: Motilal Bararsidass, 2000. First published in 1934 by Oxford University Press.

Desikachar, Kausthub. *The Yoga of the Yogi: The Legacy of T. Krishnamacharya.* Chennai (India): Krishnamacharya Yoga Mandiram, 2005.

Desikachar, T.K.V. *Health Healing and Beyond: Yoga and the Living Tradition of Krishnamacharya.* With R. H. Cravens. New York: Aperture, 1998.

———. *The Heart of Yoga: Developing a Personal Practice.* Rochester, VT: Inner Traditions International, 1995.

———. *In Search of Mind.* Chennai (India): Krishnamacharya Yoga Mandiram, 1998.

———. *Reflections on Yoga Sūtra-s of Patañjali.* 2nd edition. Chennai (India): Krishnamacharya Yoga Mandiram, 2003.

———. *Religiousness in Yoga: Lectures on Theory and Practice.* Edited by Mary Louise Skelton and John Ross Carter. Washington, DC: University Press of America, 1980.

———. *The Viniyoga of Yoga: Applying Yoga for Healthy Living.* With Kausthub Desikachar and Frans Moors. Chennai (India): Krishnamacharya Yoga Mandiram, 2001.

———. *What Are We Seeking?* With Martyn Neal. Chennai (India): Krishnamacharya Yoga Mandiram, 2001.

———, and Arjun Rajagopalan. *The Yoga of Healing.* Chennai/Bangalore/Hyderabad (India): EastWest Books, 1999.

Deussen, Paul. *Outlines of Indian Philosophy: With an Appendix on the Philosophy of the Vedânta in Its Relations to Occidental Metaphysics.* Charleston, SC: BiblioLife, 2009. First published in 1907 by Karl Curtius.

Dowson, John. *A Classical Dictionary of Hindu Mythology and Religion, Geography, History and Literature.* New Delhi: D.K. Printworld, 2000. First published in 1879 by Trübner & Co.

Freud, Sigmund. *Beyond the Pleasure Principle.* Translated and edited by James Strachey. New York: W. W. Norton, 1989. First published in German in 1920 under the title *Jenseits des Lustprinzips.*

———. *The Ego and the Id.* Translated and edited by James Strachey. New York: W. W. Norton, 1989. First published in German in 1923 under the title *Das Ich und das Es.*

———. *Five Lectures on Psycho-Analysis.* Translated and edited by James Strachey. New York: W. W. Norton, 1989. First published in German in 1910 under the title *Über Psychoanalyse: Fünf Vorlesungen.*

———. *Inhibitions, Symptoms and Anxiety.* Translated by Alix Strachey. Revised and edited by James Strachey. New York: W. W. Norton, 1989. First published in German in 1926 under the title *Hemmung, Symptom und Angst.*

———. *Introductory Lectures on Psycho-Analysis.* Translated and edited by James Strachey. New York: W. W. Norton, 1989. First published in German in 1917 under the title *Vorlesungen zur Einführung in die Psychoanalyse.*

———. *New Introductory Lectures on Psycho-Analysis.* Translated and edited by James Strachey. New York: W. W. Norton, 1989. First published in German in 1933 under the title *Neue Folge der Vorlesungen zur Einführung in die Psychoanalyse.*

———. *On Dreams.* Translated and edited by James Strachey. New York: W. W. Norton, 1989. First published in German in 1901 under the title *Über den Traum.*

———. *An Outline of Psycho-Analysis.* Translated and newly edited by James Strachey. New York: W. W. Norton, 1989. First published in German in 1938 under the title *Abriss der Psycho-Analyse.*

———. *The Psychopathology of Everyday Life.* Translated by Alan Tyson. Edited by James Strachey. New York: W. W. Norton, 1989. First published in German in 1901 under the title *Zur Psychopathologie des Alltagslebens.*

Hillebrand, Alfred, trans. *Upanishaden: Die Geheimlehre der Inder.* Düsseldorf/Cologne: Diederichs, 1979.

Iyengar, B.K.S. *Light on Prānāyāma: The Yogic Art of Breathing.* London: Allen & Unwin, 1981.

———. *Light on Yoga*. London: Allen & Unwin, 1966.

Kantrowitz, Judy L. "The Beneficial Aspects of the Patient-Analyst Match." *International Journal of Psycho-Analysis* 76 (April 1995): 299–313.

Kernberg, Otto F. *Internal World and External Reality: Object Relations Theory Applied*. New York: J. Aronson, 1980.

Klein, Melanie. *The Psycho-Analysis of Children*. Translated by Alix Strachey. Revised in collaboration with Alix Strachey by H. A. Thorner. New York: Delacorte Press/S. Lawrence, 1975.

Krishnamurti, Jiddu. *Ideal und Wirklichkeit*. Edited by Rajagpal in collaboration with Anne Vigeveno. 10th edition. Bern: Humata Verlag Harold S. Blume, 1986.

Krusche, Hellfried. "Probleme bei der Erfolgsbeurteilung von Psychoanalysen bei traumatisierten Patienten." In *Symptom—Konflikt—Struktur: Rückkehr einer alten Debatte; Psychoanalyse als Behandlungsmethode im Spannungsfeld zwischen Störungsspezifität und krankem Individuum*, edited by Sybille Drews, 279–97. Printed by the editor, 2001.

———. "Psychoanalysis." In Desikachar and Rajagopalan, *The Yoga of Healing*, 49–55.

———. "Psychothérapie, Psychanalyse et Yoga." *Viniyoga* 50 (1996).

———. *"Schade um die schöne Zeit": Zur Erfolgsbeurteilung psychoanalytischer Langzeitbehandlungen bei traumatisierten Patienten*. Kassel: Universität Gesamthochschule, 2001.

———. "Wilfred Bion zwischen fernöstlicher Mystik und westlicher Aufklärung." In *Tauchgänge*, edited by Thomas Hartung and Laura Viviana Strauss, 147–74. Göttingen: Vandenhoeck & Ruprecht, 2013.

Lear, Jonathan. "An Interpretation of Transference." *International Journal of Psycho-Analysis*, 74 (August 1993): 739–55.

Leuzinger-Bohleber, Marianne, and Ulrich Stuhr (eds.). *Psychoanalysen im Rückblick: Methoden, Ergebnisse und Perspektiven der neueren Katamneseforschung*. Gießen: Psychosozial-Verlag, 1997.

Lokeswarananda, Swami. *Taittirīya Upariṣad*. 2nd edition. Calcutta: Ramakrishna Mission Institute of Culture, 2005.

Lorelle, Christiane Berthelet. *La sagesse du désir: Le yoga et la psychanalyse*. Paris: Seuil, 2003.

Maman, Laurence, and Hellfried Krusche. *La dimension relationelle: Dans la transmission du yoga*. Sainte-Cécile-les-vignes (France): Les Cahiers de Présence d'Esprit, 2005.

Modell, Arnold H. *Other Times, Other Realities: Toward a Theory of Psychoanalytic Treatment*. Cambridge, MA: Harvard University Press, 1990.

Parthasarathy, A. *The Symbolism of Hindu Gods and Rituals*. Mumbai: Vakil & Sons, 2005. First published in 1983 by Vedanta Life Institute.

Prasāda, Rāma (trans.). *Pātañjali's Yoga Sutras*. New Delhi: Munshiram Manoharlal, 2003. First published in 1912 by Pāṇiṇi Office.

Radhakrishnan, S. (ed. and trans.). *The Principal Upaniṣads*. New Delhi: HarperCollins, 2004. First published in 1953 by Allen & Unwin.

Rajagopalachari. C. *Ramayana*. Mumbai: Bhavan's Book University, 2000. First published in 1951 by Bharatiya Vidya Bhavan.

Rukmani, T. S. *Yogasūtrabhāṣyavivaraṇa of Śaṅkara*. 2 vols. New Delhi: Munshiram Manoharlal, 2001.

Sander, Friedrich, and Hans Volkelt. *Ganzheitspsychologie*. 2nd edition, revised. Munich: C. H. Beck, 1967.

Sandler, Joseph, and Anna Ursula Dreher. *What Do Psychoanalysts Want? The Problem of Aims in Psychoanalytic Therapy*. London/New York: Routledge, 1996.

Schopenhauer, Arthur. *On the Will in Nature: A Discussion of the Corroborations from the Empirical Sciences That the Author's Philosophy Has Received Since Its First Appearance*. Translated by E.F.J. Payne. Edited by David E. Cartwright. New York/Oxford: Berg, 1992.

Smith, M.J.N. *An Illustrated Guide to Asanas and Pranayama*. Chennai (India): Krishnamacharya Yoga Mandiram, 1980.

Swarupananda, Swami. *Srimad-Bhagavad-Gita*. Calcutta: Advaita Ashrama, 1996. First published in 1909 by Advaita Ashrama.

Taimini, I. K. *Gāyatrī: The Daily Religious Practice of the Hindus*. 6th edition. Adyar/Chennai (India): Theosophical Publishing House, 1974.

Verma, Vinod. *Patañjali and Āyurvedic Yoga*. Delhi: Motilal Banarsidass Publishers, 2002.

Winnicott, D. W. *Playing and Reality*. London: Tavistock, 1971.

Zimmer, Heinrich. *Philosophies of India*. Edited by Joseph Campbell. London: Routledge & Kegan Paul, 1952.